GETTING
FIT FOR
Jesus

A six-week interactive guide to feed
the mind, body, and soul to become
your best self physically and spiritually

Meal Plans with Grocery Lists

Gluten Free Recipes

Daily Devotions

Workout Plans That Burn Fat Fast

A Chance to Grow Your Walk with God

Getting Fit for Jesus

Available from Amazon.com, CreateSpace.com, and other retail outlets

ISBN-13: 978-1981228522

ISBN-10: 1981228527

Cover design: Savannah Draper
Interior design: Savannah Smith
Editor: Abbigail Willingham
Photography: Aaron Bryant
Author: Jessi Willingham

CreateSpace, Charleston SC

Contents

To Adam

For being the godly man our family needs and
never giving up on me. I love you.

To Reed and Avery

I pray you always follow God and put Him first,
even if it means taking the road less traveled.
Momma loves you.

Prologue

To get the most out of this book I encourage you to have something to write with and a highlighter in hand. This is an interactive book that prompts you to write your thoughts and ideas into the given spaces. Highlight anything you deem important.

I want to extend a huge congratulation on taking this first step into bettering your life. You are reading this book and embarking on this journey because you are ready for a change. Maybe you are looking to shed a few pounds and tone up; maybe you are trying to eat healthier, or gluten free; or maybe you are lost and needing God's guidance through the storms in your life. If you are like me, I was looking for all the above. Sadly, in all my relentless searching I could not find a book (other than the Bible of course) that laid out an in-depth plan for what I needed to better all aspects of my life. Thus, *Getting Fit for Jesus* was born. Before I start telling you about my book I'll share a little about myself.

My name is Jessi, typically when I first meet someone they think I'm saying "J.C." because of my thick southern accent. I was raised on our family farm in rural Northwest Georgia and that is where I still reside today with my amazing husband of seven years and our two beautiful babies, my three-year old Reed and one-year old Avery Ann.

Adam and I grew up in the same county but did not start dating until I was in college. I played softball in college then decided God had other plans for my life so I began pursuing a career as an Occupational Therapy Assistant. Right after graduating I worked in a school system with special needs children, I then took a job at a hospital where I was working inpatient and outpatient rehab. It was during that time that I became pregnant (twice) and had my babies.

Having two small children is no walk in the park, most days I'm lucky to put clothes on, but the good Lord has blessed Adam and I so that I can stay at home and raise my kids and I wouldn't have it any other way.

I have always had a passion for working out and staying active. During high school and college, I would go to the gym at least once a day. Even after I started working in the real world I would still have three to four workouts in a week.

It's crazy how much your life changes when babies come into the picture. When God and family were put first in my life, going to a gym was somewhere between last and next to last on my priority list. Then a series of health issues arose and after many doctor visits and tests it turns out I have a gluten intolerance that came about after having Avery.

This was a very trying time in my life where my faith in our Lord was truly tested. But like all storms He was there by my side during the whole ordeal. That's when I felt God pulling on my heart and working in my life getting me ready to write this book. No matter the reason your reading these words know that God has a plan for your life and I hope that after reading this book, that plan becomes a little clearer for you.

Getting
STARTED

The hardest part of any life change is taking that first step… and guess what… by turning the pages in this book you have officially started climbing that mountain. It will not be easy, but my prayer for you is that you embrace all of life, good and bad, and give the glory to God in all that you do. In doing so, it's amazing at the things He can accomplish in your life. Not only is this six-week interactive book going to teach you healthy habits to help you lose weight, eat better, and feel better, but it's going to re-kindle that walk with God that He intends us to have.

There are a few essential healthy tips I want to share with you before you embark on this journey with me. Before I share with you my tips, please remember that I am not a doctor, nutritionist, or personal trainer. I am a momma that has always been mindful of my health and what I put on and in my body, so I've conducted research and figured out what works for me and my body through trial and error. You know your body better than any-one else and if I'm telling you to do something that you don't think will be beneficial, then don't do it. Check with your regular care physician before starting any exercise program to make sure you're healthy enough for that type of activity.

Everything in this book has helped me achieve the results I wanted, which was a strong and lean body. I didn't care about the scale, but about how I felt in my own skin. This is a tool to help you achieve your goals, not a fix all. I'm not going to make claims that you're going to lose 10 or 20 or 30 pounds. Everyone's body has been created differently therefore you will get out of this what you put into it. I pray that at the end of this book you have become your own body's advocate and you're able to make healthy choices yourself! I do not want people to read it one time and put it down. My goal is for people to read it, take notes, highlight, go back and re-read, write in it. Wear the cover out!

Tip number one is drink your water! I know you have heard this time and time again, however water is a huge part of your life and wellbeing. Drinking enough water aids in digestion while flushing out your kidneys, it helps reduce headaches, protects your joints by keeping them lubricated, it gives you more energy, more elastic skin, and when you are drinking enough water, you feel all around better and are less tired (and as a busy momma I am all about having more energy). My goal is to drink half of my body weight in ounces daily, for example 125lbs/2=64oz. I also drink a daily morning detox water to get my digestion started in the mornings which consists of 8oz hot water, ½ fresh squeezed lemon, and 1 tbl of apple cider vinegar.

Tip number two is to start looking and reading the labels on your food before you make a purchase. I'm not going to tell you to count carbs or only eat certain foods. Just know that it is all about balance! The number one thing that you should consider is the amount of sugar in an item. For the next six weeks, I have only included items that have 9g of sugar or less in one serving size. Processed and refined sugars are bad for your liver, teeth, and your skin. Sugar messes with your hormones and it actually sends messages to your brain telling you to eat more because it's just empty calories. There have also been studies that link sugar to cancer growth.

In my opinion, sugar is a silent killer. Just like with everything I mention in this book, don't take my word on it. Be your own advocate and do your own research to decide for yourself if you feel the same way I do about sugar. For me sugar is addicting, the more I eat sugar the more I want it. However, now that I have taken out refined sugars from my diet I no longer crave sugar like I once did. So, if you must have that brownie, have a portion size that equals 9g of sugar. Hopefully after completing these next 6 weeks you'll not want that refined sugar filled brownie and instead will be craving good whole foods or my healthy brownie recipe (that's right! It's healthy! And chocolate!!).

I am a staunch supporter of proper portion sizes and listening to your body. Which leads me to the fact that I want you to start reading and following what the serving size is on different items. If you're going to eat those crackers, don't eat half the sleeve, eat the amount that's in one serving size. This book also has meal plans for the week along with fun recipes to get in added vegetables. All the recipes are gluten free! I'm all about getting whole, real foods into your diet and drastically limiting your processed foods.

Okay, let's do a little test.

Go into your cabinet and pick out something that you use all the time. Look at the back of the label.

What is the serving size? ________________

How much sugar is in that particular serving size? ___________

Do you honestly just eat one serving size? ____________________

These are things you need to be asking yourself every time you shop at the grocery store or pull something from the pantry to cook. If this item isn't the most nutritious, what is something healthier you can substitute for it?

Tip number three is to forget every other diet you have ever been on. Literally forget them! Throw out the fad diet cookbooks, pills, and diet plans promising you'll shed 20 pounds in 20 days. Because we've all been there, and let's face it, those drastic diets may work for a season, but they all fail in the end. Why is that? Because they are not meant to be completed for the rest of our lives. They are meant to be done so you can see results in a few weeks. Then your body plateaus and you become bored with doing the same 30-minute exercise video every night. You find yourself reverting back to your old habits of eating junk food and not being active. This leaves you feeling defeated and negative towards yourself. It's a vicious cycle that will just continue unless you put a stop to it right now. This is not a diet! This is a lifestyle change.

You're going to incorporate new healthy habits in your everyday life while feeding your soul and by the end of this book you'll be equipped with the knowledge to be your own advocate! You should understand the importance of cooking fresh whole foods, exercising, and putting God first in your life. You will have an entirely different outlook on life, which will hopefully end that vicious cycle of feeling like a failure or inadequate. I will forever strive to stay tone, fit, lean, and healthy so I can keep up with my family and do God's work He's put me on this earth to do.

I've created this six-week start up guide for you to think outside the box when it comes to exercising. You will only need weights if you want to make the exercises harder, but they are not required. Also please keep in mind that your Bible is to be utilized, not idolized. Open God's word. Use the tool He has given you and just like you'd do research about your body, do research in His word about your spiritual self. Please do not replace your Bible with this book but instead use my book alongside your Bible to receive a blessing.

Tip number four, purge your kitchen! This is a biggie and hopefully after this book your kitchen, home, life, body, and soul will all be purged of the nasty junk the devil wants in your life so that your eyes are taken off God.

But I'm getting ahead of myself so let's just talk about your kitchen for a moment. As a stay at home momma, when I'm home I feel like most of the day is spent in the kitchen. I prepare three meals a day plus tons of snacks for a growing toddler, clean up the mess, and do it all over again. When I first wake up in the mornings, I sit at my kitchen island and map out my day while sipping my morning detox water and reading my devotion. If I'm going to be spending that much time in my kitchen I want it to be a welcoming, fun, inspiring place that you can go and feel energized, not bogged down because all the clutter, or nasty junk food that's going to tempt you to "fall off the wagon."

Let me ask you a question, where do you go to relax and sleep in your home? Typically, your bed, right? Because you've trained your brain to recognize that space as a place for rest. A place to shut down and recharge the batteries. What have you trained your brain and body to feel when you're in the kitchen? Over the years I've remodeled my kitchen and cleaned it out to eliminate the clutter so it's more pleasing to the eye. But the biggest overhaul was in the refrigerator and pantry. If you're truly wanting to rid your life of junk, it starts with what you are putting in your body.

When I walk into my kitchen I don't feel that need to binge eat or snack on everything I see. How, you ask? Because I have trained my brain and body to look at my kitchen as a healthy place, a fun place my family can go and open the fridge and see a rainbow of washed fruits and vegetables they can pull out and snack on anytime of day. An inspiring place where I can experiment with different recipes. A happy place that is helping me reach my goal of becoming a better me.

Go and look in your pantry. If it's a processed food with over 9g of sugar (and in my case if it has gluten) then chuck it! Donate it to a food pantry and don't look back. I hear people all the time telling me, "I'll use it up then I just won't buy it again." For those of you who have a hard time throwing out food (which I totally get and respect) I say this, what if you used a laundry soap that gave you an itchy red rash, would you use it up till it was gone then try to fix the rash? Of course not! It's doing damage to your body. The foods you are putting into your system, if not good for you, are harming your bodies from the inside out. You only get one body so why would you intentionally do it harm? Throw out the junk food right now! Don't wait! Remember the hardest part was taking that first step of opening this book, and you already rocked it! So now take this next step and fully commit to this six weeks of getting fit for Jesus! You will not be disappointed.

Finally, tip number five is to take the survey you'll find on the next page. I urge you to dig down deep and be brutally honest with yourself. There is also another survey at the end of this book that you will be doing to see your progress. This book alongside your Bible is what I hope will help you get closer to God while getting a healthy body. I am a huge believer in the holistic approach to your health. You must feed your body, mind, and soul. This book has that and I can't wait for us to begin your healthy lifestyle change.

To recap on everything we just discussed you need to drink water, start reading your labels for nutrition information, look for items with 9g of sugar or less, forget your past diets and get it the right head space to begin this journey, purge your kitchen, and take the survey.

Survey
BEFORE STARTING THE Program

This is just a baseline to see where you're at in your life spiritually, physically, and emotionally. Please do this during a quiet time when you have limited distractions so you can be honest with yourself and take your time. Remember, God already knows how you feel, the question is are you ready to admit it to yourself.

Age:

Height:

Weight:

What are you looking to get out of this six-week program concerning your body? (i.e. lose weight, walk up the stairs without feeling the need to faint or vomit etc.)

What are you looking to get out of this six-week program concerning your spiritual life? (i.e. closer walk with God, creating a habit to complete a devotion with prayer every day, I don't know if I am even a Christian etc.)

Circle the best answer that describes you at this time:

When I think of food…
A)   I think about how God made it as fuel for my body
B)   I feel like I have an eating disorder
C)   I get depressed because I know it will only turn to fat
D)   I must be stressed
E)   I think maybe it will make me happy if I eat something
F)   Other: ______________________________

When I think about working out…
a)   I think it's only for skinny people who are already in shape
b)   I don't think I have time
c)   I don't- I don't enjoy working out
d)   I feel like it gives me energy to accomplish Gods work
e)   I sort of feel like working out because I know it's good for me
f)   Other: ______________________________

My walk with God is…
a)   Struggling
b)   Non-existent
c)   Strained, I don't give him the time He deserves
d)   Great
e)   Better than it once was
f)   Other: ______________________________

Write out 3 short term goals you want to achieve within this 6 weeks
1.   ______________________________
2.   ______________________________
3.   ______________________________

Write out 3 long term goals (year or longer) you wish to achieve after reading this book
1.   ______________________________
2.   ______________________________
3.   ______________________________

Prioritize the following, 1 being most important in your life right now and 15 being least important:

___financial wealth
___family
___friends, my social status
___God
___working out
___eating a well-balanced diet
___my spouse
___my career
___my car
___my house
___my prayer life
___how others see me
___how I look
___how I feel
___my clothes

Picture time! Take a picture of the front of your body, side view, back view, and then of a cute pose. Make it fun! And make them all full body shots. Take them right now and then you will take pictures again at the end of the six-weeks to see your results!

Now for a short fitness test. Put 30 seconds on a stop watch and see how many squats, pushups, and crunches you can do in the allotted amount of time.

30 seconds of squats _____________
30 seconds of pushups _______________
30 seconds of crunches _______________

All done!!!! Yay!!! That wasn't that bad, was it?

Lord God, Your omnipotent love is deep. You know I am scared, excited, and ready to begin this six-week challenge to not only better myself on the outside, but on the inside. I give you all the credit and glory. Help others see the change happening in my life and let your light shine through me so that others may be led to you as well. Give me the strength to persevere when it gets hard and when the devil tempts me. I love you and thank you for all your many blessings. In Jesus' name. Amen.

Program OVERVIEW

This program has six weeks of meal plan ideas along with workouts to help you get you that toned, lean, strong body you've always wanted. The workouts get harder as the weeks progress, but fear not, the workouts have been made to where you can make the exercises as easy or as hard as you want. The results you acquire from the program will be based on how much effort you put into following the meal plans and workouts!

Here's a rundown of the workouts for the next six weeks:

	Mon	Tues	Wed	Thurs	Fri	Sat	Sun
Week 1	HD		L		HD	FD	PY
Week 2	HD		L		HD	FD	PY
Week 3	HD	L		HD	L	FD	PY
Week 4	HD	L		HD	L	FD	PY
Week 5	HD	L	HD	YC*	HD	FD	PY
Week 6	HD	L	HD	YC*	HD	FD	PY-YC*

HD- hum dingers: These will be your favorite days, not because they're easy any means, but because you're going to burn a ton of fat doing these fun, fast pace workouts. You are guaranteed to sweat on these days!

L- light days: Don't let the name of these days fool you, you're still going to get a great workout in if you give it your all. However, these workouts are designed to stretch your body and keep it moving while keeping you lean and strong, not bulky.

FD- fitness dares! These are my favorite! Every Saturday it takes your fitness routine and turns it upside down. These days will get you out of your comfort zone and help you realize that you don't have to have a gym membership or be away from your family to get in a great workout that is not only challenging, but a lot of fun. It gets you outside in God's beautiful creation and gets you thinking about how much more life has to offer. You will find six FD's starting on page 91. You will choose one of those FD's to plug into every Saturday for six weeks. I encourage you to attempt all six of these FD's… I dare you!

PY- pamper yourself! We tend to forget ourselves in our hectic busy life. However, Sundays are supposed to be a time for fellowship, family, and we can't forget ourselves. God gave us Sundays so we as humans had a day to slow down and remember Jesus Christ our Lord and Savior that paid the ultimate sacrifice so we could have an eternal home in heaven. We need to thank God daily for this, but especially on Sundays. You will not have a workout on Sunday but instead, little DIY activities for you to treat yourself and get in the right mindset for the upcoming week. What you'll be doing on the PY days:

Week one: DIY hair mask

Week two: Sugar body scrub

Week three: Oil pulling for teeth

Week four: DIY face mask

Week five: Paint your nails

Week six: YC* pamper day, pick the one you liked the most or come up with something on your own.

YC*- Your Choice: These days are super special. The whole purpose of this book is to give yourself the confidence to be the best you that you can be, while creating a new healthy lifestyle. That means once this six-week program is finished you need to have a plan about what you're going to do from there. We've already talked about that vicious cycle we are trying to get away from so by making you choose different aspects of your healthy life plan towards the end of the six weeks, it will allow you to think for yourself and create additional healthy habits that work for your busy schedule that will last a lifetime.

Week One

Meal Plan

Here's an overview of the week. First let's look at your meal plan and grocery list...

	Breakfast	Snack 1	Lunch	Snack 2	Supper
Monday	Turmeric Oatmeal*	Carrots and Hummus	Chef Salad*	Blueberries and Walnuts	Stuffed Peppers*
Tuesday	Loaded Omelet*	Cheese Stick	Stuffed Pepper Leftovers	Apple	Very Veggie Spaghetti*
Wednesday	Chocolate Smoothie*	Blueberries and Walnuts	Spaghetti Leftovers	Carrots and Hummus	Chicken Caesar Salad*
Thursday	Turmeric Oatmeal	Apple	Chicken Caesar Salad Leftovers	Cheese Stick	Shrimp Scampi Pasta*
Friday	Loaded Omelet	Carrots and Hummus	Shrimp Scampi Pasta Leftovers	Blueberries and Walnuts	BBQ with Broccoli Slaw*
Saturday	Chocolate Smoothie	Cheese Stick	BBQ Leftovers	Apple	Chicken Avacado Burritos*
Sunday	Pancakes, Eggs, Bacon (aka Willingham Family Tradition)	Blueberries and Walnuts	Chicken Avocado Leftovers	Carrots and Hummus	Eat Out

*There are recipes for these meals starting on page 95. There are also some very tasty healthy desserts!

Grocery List

SPICES
TURMERIC
HONEY
CACAO POWDER
COCONUT OIL
CINNAMON
LIQUID STEAK SEASONING
WORCESTERSHIRE SAUCE
DRIED BAY LEAVES
GROUND MUSTARD
CELERY SEED
APPLE CIDER VINEGAR (ACV)
RANCH DRESSING
CAESAR DRESSING
CHICKEN STOCK
16 OZ. SPAGHETTI SAUCE

PRODUCE
MUSHROOMS
PEPPERS (5)
SPINACH
BANANAS
ZUCCHINI (1)
STRAWBERRIES
ICEBERG LETTUCE
ROMAINE LETTUCE
BAG OF CARROTS
AVOCADO (1)
HUMMUS
10 0Z DICED TOMATOES
WITH PEPPERS
80Z TOMATO JUICE
ONION (2)
GARLIC
BAG FROZEN BROCCOLI
LEMONS
BAG OF APPLES
BAG OF BROCCOLI SLAW

PROTEIN
FLAX SEED
PEANUT BUTTER (OR ANY
NUT BUTTER)
EGGS
CUBED HAM
CHIA SEEDS
DELI MEAT (TURKEY)
BACON
WALNUTS
12 OZ. ITALIAN SAUSAGE
1 LB. GROUND BEEF
2 PACKS CHICKEN BREAST
BAG OF FROZEN SHRIMP
1-2 LB. DEER ROAST (OR
MEAT OF CHOICE)

DAIRY
ALMOND MILK
CHEDDAR CHEESE
SHREDDED MOZZARELLA
CHEESE
CHEESE STICKS
PARMESAN CHEESE

GRAINS
OLD FASHION OATS
CORN TORTILLAS
GLUTEN FREE (GF) PANCAKE
MIX
BROWN RICE
GF SPAGHETTI NOODLES
GF SPIRAL NOODLES

*** BEFORE CREATING YOUR WEEKLY GROCERY LISTS, I ENCOURAGE YOU TO LOOK AT THE WEEKLY MEAL PLANNER AND THEN GO IN THE BACK OF THE BOOK TO LOOK AT THE RECIPE. YOU MAY FIND THAT YOU WANT TO ADD OR TAKE AWAY SOMETHING FROM A RECIPE OR FROM THE WEEK IN GENERAL. THIS IS A GUIDELINE ONLY. YOUR FAMILY SIZE WILL ALSO DETERMINE HOW MUCH OF SOMETHING YOU NEED. TAKE ALL THIS INTO CONSIDERATION BEFORE HEADING OUT TO THE STORE.

Monday, Devotion 1- Cup Size

"I will praise thee; for I am fearfully and wonderfully made: marvelous are thy works: and that my soul knoweth right well." Psalm 139: 14 KJV

"You made all the delicate, inner parts of my body and knit me together in my mother's womb. Thank you for making me so wonderfully complex! Your workmanship is marvelous how well I know it." Psalm 139:13-14 NLT Study Bible

When I was a little girl, I was very much a tomboy. I would hang with the guys and get in the mud well before going inside and playing dress up or dolls with the girls. I would even cry when my mom made me put on a dress for church! However, once I got into middle school I began putting on makeup, trying (and typically failing) to fix my hair, and looking at myself and sadly comparing myself to the other girls who were, "well endowed". I am now 27 years old and I am barely an A cup. Let's face it, bras with Barbie and Disney characters on them fit me better than an adult bra. But because a grown woman shopping in the junior department for a bra is a little silly I typically stick to sports bras.

I can now laugh at my past insecurities and know that is just how God made me. However, that wasn't always the case. Kids are mean, and I would find myself in a lot of my "friend's" jokes. So why did this bother me? Sin. I began comparing myself to others and quickly forgetting what the Bible teaches in Psalms. God created me, He formed me in my mother's womb and knew exactly how I was going to look. So why, knowing that God is perfect and He doesn't make mistakes, would I be upset or want to change my physical appearance by having cosmetic surgery? Knowing God made me this way. I am not bashing those that have had surgery to change their appearances, but for me, I feel God wants me to use my past insecurity to show young girls out there that you are beautiful just the way you are.

What are you insecure about?

Thank God for creating you just like you are and know that He loves you.

How can you use your insecurities to help others?

Thank you Heavenly Father for making me just the way I am! Please help me to embrace my insecurities and use that in a way to help be a witness to someone who also has insecurities. Help me use my body for your service. In Jesus' name. Amen.

***HD #1 is the workout for the day. You'll find this exercises on page 81.

Tuesday, Devotion 2- Change for the Better

"And he said unto his disciples, therefore I say unto you, take no thought for your life, what ye shall eat; neither for the body, what ye shall put on. The life is more than meat and the body is more than raiment." Luke 12:22-23 KJV

"Then turning to his disciples, Jesus said, that is why I tell you not to worry about everyday life-whether you have enough food to eat or enough clothes to wear. For life is more than food, and your body more than clothing." Luke 12:22-23 NLT Study Bible

My ten-year high school reunion is coming up next year! At times, I can't believe it has been that long since I stood in front of my graduating peers and delivered the class president speech, wishing them happiness and prosperity in all they do. When I talk to other people about high school days this statement always pops up somewhere in our conversation, "I wish I looked now like I did back then." I totally get wanting to look your best and walking into your class reunion (or anywhere of importance) and all the jaws drop at how good you look with your slim and trim physique and your awesome wardrobe! We've all had that daydream once or twice, but is that the reason why you're working out and wanting a lifestyle change? To show other people how accomplished you are or how young you look? Are you putting your fitness and appearances before your family, before Christ?

If these types of thoughts are running through your mind when you're thinking about the reasons you are wanting to change your habits and get healthy I urge you to stop, and dive into the word of God. He tells us in His great book that there's more to life than food, clothing, and appearances. If you are trying to change your looks because you want to make some other woman jealous, or a man look at you in a sexual way then you're doing my six-week program for all the wrong reasons. Change your body to honor the Lord. Have a strong body and use that body and gifts God has given you to further His kingdom. Do it to show your children, peers, and loved ones that living a healthy life for Christ doesn't mean you must follow the latest fashion trends or be supermodel skinny. It means being the best YOU that YOU can be and that means putting Christ first, not fitness.

We can easily get wrapped up in the social stigma of having to look good all the time. But that all fades away and people will forget what you wore. But how you live for Christ… that will last for eternity. That's what I hope people will see in me when I go to my class reunion next year.

What do you want others to see in you?

Who are you changing your life for? How can this change in you help further God's kingdom?

Heavenly Father, please rid me of the vain thoughts and instead fill me with an urge to better myself to further your Kingdom. Amen.

Rest Day!!! Enjoy!

Wednesday, Devotion 3- Sleeping Baby

"And the LORD, he it is that doith go before thee; he will be with thee, he will not fail thee, neither forsake thee: fear not, neither be dismayed." Deuteronomy 31:8 KJV

"Do not be afraid or discouraged, for the LORD will personally go ahead of you. He will be with you; he will neither fail you nor abandon you." Deuteronomy 31:8 NLT Study Bible

If you're a parent then you'll understand me when I say that my body, once requiring at least eight hours of sleep, can now somehow function with three hours of sleep and waking up all hours of the night. Nothing good has ever come out of me being awake at 4am, however, it was in an ordinary, sleepy moment at 4am when I was attempting (and failing) to rock my then four-month-old son back to sleep when God spoke to me. I remember being so tired that night. I was rocking my son in his dimly lit room silently begging him to go back to sleep. I was trying to cuddle him close to me because his eyes were closed and he was relentlessly reaching and searching for me. However, he was reaching the wrong way! I was just sitting there watching him silently pleading with him to just turn his head and reach his arms the other way so he would feel my warm embrace and fall back to sleep. I then thought about that must be how our heavenly Father feels all the time.

We as humans want to handle things on our own and in our time, we feel as if God isn't there and we're searching and searching, but just can't seem to find the peace we are looking for. God, just like me sitting there in my chair that night, doesn't move. He has never left us and He's holding us in His all-mighty embrace and He is begging us to just relax and cast our cares on Him because He has always been there. It is US that grow farther away from God.

Are you searching for something on your own because you feel as if God just isn't there?

I encourage you to remember that He will neither fail you nor abandon you. He is just waiting on us to finally let go and turn back to Him.

Father, You know my heart and you know that I have been trying to handle _____________ on my own. Please let me give it to You and turn back into Your embrace. Thank you Lord for everything you do for me and my family. Amen.

L #1 is your workout for today. It's located on page 87, you've got this!

Thursday, Devotion 4- Mississippi Money

"For the wages of sin is death; but the gift of God is eternal life through Jesus Christ our Lord." Romans 6:23 KJV

"For the wages of sin is death, but the free gift of God is eternal life through Christ Jesus our Lord." Romans 6:23 NLT Study Bible

I have some of the fondest memories of my brother and I spending a week at my grandparents' house in Pope, Mississippi. My PawPaw is a Southern Baptist preacher and every summer we would plan our trip based on when his church was having their Vacation Bible School. I will never forget the final night's lesson he gave one very hot Mississippi summer night. He gathered all the children up in the sanctuary and he pulled out of his pocket a 20-dollar bill. Now my grandparents always took us to a dime store downtown and we thought we were something because they gave us one whole crisp dollar to purchase something from that store. So, when he pulled that twenty-dollar bill out of his pocket I immediately got excited! Think of all those stick-on earrings and bubble gum I could buy with that bad boy!

When all attention was directed on my PawPaw he said, "This twenty bucks is free to the first person that comes up and grabs it." It happened so fast, yet it was like I was watching in slow motion all the kids around me. Some jumped up and ran as fast as they could to my PawPaw. Others' reflexes were either terribly slow or they were second guess-ing whether or not they should leave their seat and attempt to elbow their way through the crowd that was already accumulating. Some never seemed to move a muscle and just sat with their arms crossed. My gut response was to jump up and run over to him and pull the whole, "I'm your granddaughter therefore I'm more entitled than the other kids," but I just sat on the pew, I let my mind get the better of me and started thinking how this was too good to be true. Why would he give away a perfectly good 20-dollar bill to some random kid, he probably wants us to do something before he gives it to us. So I didn't go up there. And some other kid grabbed that 20 bucks and went and sat down. PawPaw didn't ask anything of him and I was feeling completely in shock that the boy who grabbed the money just took it and didn't earn it at all!! PawPaw then shared an amazing lesson with us all. He told us that God has a gift for us also. It's free for those who believe and take it.

Have you received the Lord God's free gift of eternal salvation?

If not, go to the very back of this book on page 109 to discover the Roman Road to Salvation.

Father, You know my heart and you know what I need to do. Please help me to openly receive your free gift and help me to share how to obtain that gift with others. Amen.

Rest Day!

Friday, Devotion 5- Pickles

"No man can serve two masters; for either he will hate the one, and love the other; or else he will hold to the one, and despise the other. Ye cannot serve God and mammon." Matthew 6: 24 KJV

"No one can serve two masters. For you will hate one and love the other; you will be devoted to one and despise the other. You cannot serve both God and money." NLT Study Bible

      Every summer of my adult life I've canned cucumbers I grow from my garden and make pickles. Believe it or not, there is an art to canning those delicious pickles. Before you can put the pickling juice and spices into the jar you first must put the pickles in a particular order so you can pack as many cucumbers in as possible. If you put the juice in first, then try to put cucumbers into the jar, you're going to make a mess and have pickle juice everywhere with very few cucumbers in your jar.

      The same can be said about life. After you put God, your spouse, your children, and then other family first you will find that you still have time for the other luxuries of your life, they just won't take up all the room. If you don't have your priorities together and put things like appearances, money, careers, etc. into you jar of life first, then there will be no room for what's most important.

What are you making important today?

Father, Help me to prioritize what's most important in my life and not become consumed in the superficial stuff. Help me to show the people that I love the most that they are more important than anything this world has to offer. Thank you for blessing me with another beautiful day! Amen.

HD #2 on page 82, these exercises get harder but I know you can do it!

Saturday, Devotion 6- Who Has Your Back

"THE LORD is my light and my salvation; whom shall I fear? The LORD is the strength of my life; of who shall I be afraid?" Psalm 27:1 KJV

"The LORD is my light and my salvation-so why should I be afraid? The LORD is my fortress, protecting me from danger." Psalm 27:1 NLT Study Bible

After I had my second child I knew things were different. I'm a huge believer that if you listen to your body it will tell you when something is wrong. And something just wasn't right. After going to countless appointments and running many tests, a diagnosis was still foggy and nothing concrete. Words like cancer began popping up when I would go to see specialists. When faced with a scary situation such as potentially having cancer, we as humans immediately begin thinking of the worst. Why wouldn't we? Cancer is a very scary thing that could potentially lead to death. And if you don't have Christ as your Lord and Savior, dying is an absolute nightmare. Yet Christians do not have to fear the grave, it has been beaten! Because Jesus Christ paid the ultimate sacrifice.

If you are going through a hard time in your life where your facing a decline in health, financial problems, relationship problems, or anything that is scaring you and keeping you up at night, I want to give you words of encouragement from Psalms, it tells us not to be afraid, because the Lord is our light and our salvation.

I found out I had a gluten intolerance. I had never been allergic to anything in my entire life and now a doctor was telling me I had to completely cut out gluten from my diet (which was in absolutely everything I was eating). So yet again I was looking to God to help me get through this hurdle in my life. But I have no fear of what is to come because I know whose got my back.

Is there something scaring you today?

Father, You know that I have been really struggling with ______________ . I'm fearful and nervous and I ask that you take away my fear and anxiety and help me to remember that I am Yours and You will take care of me. Amen.

This is your first FD!!! So exciting! Go to page 91 and choose between one of the FD to perform on this day. Don't be afraid to go after it.

Sunday, Devotion 7- I'm Done

"And let us not be weary in well doing: for in due season we shall reap, if we faint not." Galatians 6:9 KJV

"So let's not get tired of doing what is good. At just the right time we will reap a harvest of blessing if we don't give up." Galatians 6:9 NLT Study Bible

Have you ever felt "over it"? I know I certainly have… over being nice, over trying to be the Godly person when everyone else seems to not care, over trying to better my body, over the whole eating good food, over not eating junk food, over working out… When I'm "over it" I look to Galatians. It tells us not to grow weary because in God's time (not ours) we will reap a harvest. For those that are feeling tired and maybe not wanting to continue your climb to betterment, keep going!

What are you over today?

Find a friend you can talk to about things that will help lift you up. Also, talk to God about your problems.

Lord, Thank you for your provisions and giving us the Bible so I can read your words when times get hard. This week I am over _________________, please help me be uplifted by Your words. Help me keep them close to my heart as I continue with the week, and with this six-week program. Amen.

PY day 1- DIY hair mask

You'll need very minimal ingredients to make this magical hair mask, I do it all the time to help my hair become softer and shinier. You'll need 4 tbl honey and 4 tbl coconut oil. Mix together (may have to microwave if the coconut oil isn't melted), massage all through hair, pull up with a clip, put a disposable shower cap on, and go relax for 15 minutes. Then just jump in the shower and wash hair like normal. Taking this little bit of time for yourself will help you feel pampered and hopefully rejuvenated for the upcoming week.

Week Two

Meal Plan

	Breakfast	Snack 1	Lunch	Snack 2	Supper
Monday	Scrambled Eggs and Blue-Bana (B-B) Muffins*	Orange	Chef Salad	Popcorn	Shepherd's Pie*
Tuesday	Strawberry Banana Smoothie*	Edamame	Shepherd's Pie Leftovers	Banana	Baked Salmon*, Steamed Broccoli, and Rice
Wednesday	Boiled Egg Sausage and Honey Toast*	Popcorn	Salmon Broccoli and Rice Leftovers	Banana	Taco Salad*
Thursday	Eggs and B-B Muffins	Orange	Taco Salad Leftovers	Popcorn	Turkey Chili*
Friday	Strawberry Banana Smoothie	Edamame	Turkey Chili Leftovers	Banana	Chef Salad
Saturday	Boiled Egg Sausage and Honey Toast	Banana	Chef Salad Leftovers	Orange	Chicken and Vegetables*
Sunday	Willingham Tradition	Orange	Chicken and Vegetables Leftovers	Popcorn	Eat Out

** The grocery list may seem like a lot for this week, but you should have a lot of the ingredients already in the pantry from where you bought them last week. Look at the recipes and the grocery list to make sure you're not buying extra. Also don't forget there are recipes in the back starting on page 95 for those meal options that containing an *

Grocery List

SPICES

HONEY
COCONUT OIL
CINNAMON
VANILLA
BAKING POWDER
BAKING SODA
SEA SALT
CHILI POWDER
CUMIN POWDER
PAPRIKA
GROUND MUSTARD
BEEF STOCK
WORCESTERSHIRE SAUCE
ACV
TACO SEASONING
RANCH DRESSING

PRODUCE

BANANA (2 BUNDLES)
APPLE SAUCE
BLUEBERRIES
ORANGES
LETTUCE
SPINACH

CARROTS
BELL PEPPER
2 SMALL ONIONS
TOMATO PASTE- 2 SMALL CANS
1 CAN TOMATO SAUCE
STRAWBERRIES (FRESH OR FROZEN)
11OZ BAG FROZEN MIXED VEGETABLES
GARLIC
POTATOES
FRESH VEGETABLE OF YOUR CHOICE (SEE ROASTED VEGETABLE RECIPE PG. 00)
EDAMAME
FROZEN BAG OF BROCCOLI
LEMONS
SALSA

PROTEIN

EGGS
WALNUTS
CANADIAN BACON
CHICKEN BREAST

DELI MEAT
2- 1 LB. GROUND BEEF
1 LB. GROUND TURKEY
1 CAN KIDNEY BEANS
1 CAN CHILI BEANS
PEANUT BUTTER
SALMON FILLETS
SAUSAGE

DAIRY

MILK
CHEDDAR CHEESE
SOUR CREAM
ALMOND MILK
BUTTER

GRAINS

GF PANCAKE MIX
GF FLOUR
POPCORN (THE REAL STUFF NOT FROM A BAG)
BROWN RICE
GF SANDWICH BREAD
TORTILLA CHIPS
OATS
CHIA SEEDS

Monday, Devotion 8- Caught in the Act

"But of that day and that hour knoweth no man, no, not the angels which are in heaven, neither the Son, but the Father." Mark 13:32 KJV

"However, no one knows the day or hour when these things will happen, not even the angels in heaven or the Son himself. Only the Father knows." Mark 13:32 NLT Study Bible

Have you ever wondered about when Christ comes back? There are many false prophets out there today saying they know the exact day when He is to return. Scripture however tells us that nobody knows, not even Jesus, when He is coming back. But when He does return, what will He find us doing? Will we be trying to lead others to Christ by loving them, praying for them, reading scripture? Or will we be drunk at a party? Fighting with a loved one? Ignoring the Holy Spirit when He's telling us to help that stranger? Following the crowd instead of standing out for Christ? Or gossiping about our co-worker?

What do you want God to find you doing when He comes back?

Father, I know that I don't always do what I'm supposed to. I know that I so often disappoint You, but please forgive me and help me to learn from my past mistakes and please give me the strength to do the right thing when it is so difficult to do so. Amen.

HD #1 on page 81, how exciting to know you've already killed this workout before. It should be easier this time around.

Tuesday, Devotion 9- Extraordinary Job

"And whatsoever ye do in word or deed, do all in the name of the Lord Jesus, giving thanks to God and the Father by him." Colossians 3:17 KJV

"And whatever you do or say, do it as a representative of the Lord Jesus, giving thanks through him to God the Father." NLT Study Bible

Careers are important to us. To some, they define who we are as a person. I had to go to school for several years, work very hard to be one of the top of my class. I was good at what I did and I was helping people get back to their lives after a stroke, heart attack, car accident or other injury had broken their bodies. Let's be honest, I felt that my job was important for the betterment of lives and I took it very seriously. Once I had my beautiful babies I felt God was leading me to stay home and raise my kiddos, but it was an adjustment. Ever since I was thirteen I worked a job. I found myself in those first months of not having a paycheck regularly coming in feeling like I was not doing my part for my family. Like I was not helping my husband out with bills. I was no longer a healthcare provider. I was just an ordinary stay at home momma. My day consisted of changing diapers, feedings, nap time where I would hopefully get a load of laundry going (not folded), more diapers and then finally after bath time and a sleepless night I'd do it all over again. I was no longer in the spotlight, and it for sure wasn't a platform for Christ. I had an ordinary job and an ordinary life (or so I thought).

Then one morning I was doing my daily devotional and I came across this verse and it was amazing at how it spoke to me. If you get nothing from this book other than this, please listen. Everything we do, if it's done for Christ, no matter how small, has an eternal impact. No, I am not working in the hospital anymore. Instead I'm working in my very own home, teaching my kids the importance of fellowship with God and what a Godly woman looks like. I am a mother, a wife, a prayer warrior, a child of God. Every day that I pray, or teach a life lesson to my children about our Lord or just call someone up and listen to what's going on in their lives, I am furthering God's kingdom and making a difference. Your job matters and whatever season of life you're in right now, know that you can make a difference. No matter how old or young, no matter how educated or uneducated, your so called ordinary life becomes extraordinary the day you decide to start living for Jesus instead of yourself.

Do you have an extraordinary life?

Father, Thank You for another day to glorify Your name. I praise Your name for reminding me today with the scripture that no matter what the world labels me, I am special, and I hold a special place in furthering Your kingdom. Amen.

Ah, Rest Day- if you are sore try some light stretching to break up the lactic acid in your body.

Wednesday, Devotion 10- God 1 Devil 0

"Thou shalt not be afraid for the terror by night; nor for the arrow that flieth by day." Psalm 91:5 KJV

"Do not be afraid of the terrors of the night, nor the arrow that flies in the day." Psalm 91:5 NLT Study Bible

It has taken me a very long time to write this book. I knew the Lord was working in my life and wanting me to do something, however when my dream got too big, it was fear that made me turn away and talk myself out of writing. Fear of rejection, failure, messing up, not getting published. Time and time again, when I heard God telling me to write this book, the devil would be very quick to try to discourage me and talk me out of it.

Fear is one of the devil's largest tools he uses to get us out of the will of God. Sometimes God asks a lot out of us, and instead of just jumping in and doing it, we over-think it and become scared of what will happen IF… I'm here to tell you today, not one time does the Bible say to fear the devil. God has already conquered the devil, He's won the war with Satan so we should not fear him. He is merely a defeated foe.

Is God asking you to do something you are afraid of?

Do you have a dream you feel is just too big to accomplish?

Lord God, Thank You for defeating the devil, he does not have a hold on me because my eyes are on You. I am scared of ___________________________, but I know that You will be with me every step of the way. Thank You for loving me no matter what. Amen.

L #1 workout on page 87.

Thursday, Devotion 11- Nutella Anyone?

"My soul shall be satisfied as with marrow and fatness; and my mouth shall praise thee with joyful lips." Psalm 63:5 KJV

"You satisfy me more than the richest feast. I will praise you with songs of joy." Psalm 63:5 NLT Study Bible

Have you ever had an extremely stressful day and the only thing you can think about is eating the whole jar of Nutella with a spoon? Yep, we've all been guilty of stress eating. Not being able to think or function until we curb our sweet tooth with some sugar. Hoping that after we down that 8oz jar of chocolate goodness we'll feel better. But sadly, we typically feel worse, because not only do we have a stomachache, but our problems didn't go away. We tried to handle them and help ourselves feel better instead of looking to God for help.

What does the Bible tell us about stress eating? It says that if we praise the Lord and give Him the glory He rightfully deserves it's better than any feast we could ever eat! Next time you're feeling like you're stressed and must eat that whole jar of Nutella, remember that your problems are not too big for God and He wants you to give them to Him. Give Him the praise instead of going for the sugar to try and fix the stress yourself.

What makes you stressed?

What's your favorite sugar indulgence? Try finding a healthier alternative, there are several dessert recipes in this book that have limited sugar, yet are still sweet and yummy.

Heavenly Father, You are the King of Kings and Lord of Lords. I lay all my burdens down at Your feet today. I no longer want to hold on to them and stress. Help me to overcome and to be lifted up so that I can lift up others. Amen.

Rest Day!

Friday, Devotion 12 – Taking Out the Trash

"And whatsoever ye do, do it heartily, as to the Lord, and not unto men." Colossians 3:23 KJV

"Work willingly at whatever you do, as though you were working for the Lord rather than for people." Colossians 3: 23 NLT Study Bible

I read something a while back that said your house is an outward representation of how you are feeling on the inside. If your house is cluttered and in a disarray, then you are more likely to feel like your life is also in a disarray. While this isn't the case with everyone, it is most definitely the case with me. I cannot function to the best of my abilities when my house is a mess. And when I'm not my best it impacts my motivation to be happy for my kids, husband, and God. I become overwhelmed and find myself having a pity party. It is so frustrating to clean all the time when a new mess is made every ten seconds. When my motivation wavers, I'm reminded that whatever I'm doing I need to do it like I was working for God. And essentially, I am, because when my house (and fridge) is cleared of junk then my mind is as well. And I can focus more on what's important like taking time for myself to get fit, having fun with my kiddos, and doing a daily devotion.

Are you in a rut and know you need to clean up your house and mind? Here are a few tips to help you get started:

Number 1: Take a trash bag and go around your whole house just throwing away trash. Old receipts, broken toys, expired foods, anything that needs thrown away.

Number 2: Quickly (being the key word) look around your house and find 15 items to donate. Yes, 15 items you no longer like in your house, or something you've stuffed into the closet and haven't used in a year, or even that cute sweater that you wore and washed one time and now it's too short. If you're not using it or are not in love with it anymore, then put it in a donatation box.

Number 3: Because most of us can't donate our things that same day, get the box out of your house. I've found myself getting such a box of donated items together but then I put it on the dining room table or floor by the door and it drives me crazy because it still looks like a cluttered mess. After you have found your 15 items, put the box in the car and get it out of your house!

Number 4: Have a timer set for 30 minutes and start making it a habit to clean non-stop for only 30 minutes a day. This will make it easier on yourself when you need to deep clean.

I find these tips to greatly help me with my cleaning routine, while keeping me motivated and not overwhelmed. Remember when you purge your house, life, and mind, you are freeing up more room for God.

What could you "clean up" in your life other than your house?

Father, Please help me to clean up all aspects of my life. Some things will be harder than others to get rid of such as bad habits like ____________, but I know with You all things are possible. Thank You for that eternal hope. Amen.

HD #2 get ready to sweat! Page 88.

Saturday, Devotion 13- Smell the Roses

"Be patient therefore, brethren, unto the coming of the Lord. Behold, the husbandman waiteth for the precious fruit of the earth, and hath long patience for it, until he receive the early and latter rain." James 5:7 KJV

"Dear brothers and sisters, be patient as you wait for the Lord's return. Consider the farmers who patiently wait for the rains in the fall and in the spring. They eagerly look for the valuable harvest to ripen." James 5:7 NLT Study Bible

We, as a society, are so impatient; instead of writing a letter, we text or e-mail, which gets it to the recipient in literally half a second. Instead of cooking a meal we run through a drive thru because we are in a rush to be somewhere. Instead of diet and exercises, we want to take a pill to become skinny fast. We even have devices now that skip all commercials on the television so we can hurry and get back to our show. With everything readily available to us right then without any wait time we naturally expect God to be the same way. But what if God's timing is different than your own? What if we have prayed for something for years and He hasn't answered us? The Bible tells us to be patient. Over the years I have learned that for me, part of my faith is having patience. Sometimes God gives us exactly what we need when we need it and it's so easy to give Him praise when that happens. It's true faith, however, when we can praise Him even when we don't get what we want right when we want it.

I challenge you all today to slow down and have a little patience, enjoy the little things we so often forget about. The rising sun, the laughter of our children, the time spent with loved ones. Even your journey of become fit, lean, and healthy. It is with this slowing down and having a little more patience is when we will find we get closer to God.

Is there something you are being impatient about today? In the space below draw a picture of your brain and what it looks like when you are stressed. Next draw your brain when you've taken the time to be patient and slow down.

Father, Your timing is never wrong and forever perfect. I thank You for the opportunities and blessings that you have, and will, bestow on me. Amen.

FD #2!!!!

Yay! Go over to page 91 and pick out which dare you want to do today. Don't forget to get the whole family involved. Helpful tip: when you're planning your meals for the week also plan your FD that way if you have to travel or let the family know to clear their schedule so everyone can go together it won't be a last minute thing.

Sunday, Devotion 14- That's my Boy

"If thou see the ass of him that hateth thee lying under his burden, and wouldest forbear to help him, thou shalt surely help with him." Exodus 23: 5 KJV

"If you see that the donkey of someone who hates you has collapsed under its load, do not walk by. Instead, stop and help." Exodus 23: 5 NLT Study Bible

My husband and I have been trying to teach my two-year-old the importance of sharing with his peers. And of course, in typical two-year-old fashion he seems to not listen to anything we are saying. Then last Sunday in nursery I watched him playing with anther little boy and he gave up his toy train so the other little boy could play with it. I honestly thought my heart was going to burst with pride! I was so proud of Reed for doing the right thing! And the best part was that I didn't have to tell him to share with that little boy. There was nothing that could take the wind out of my sails that day, and I literally wanted to go find everyone I knew and tell them "see that little boy sharing... that's my boy!"

Can't you just imagine God looking down on us feeling that same sense of pride and joy when we do the right thing here on Earth? The Holy Spirit lets us know what we should do time and time again; yet time and time again we brush Him off and take the easy route in life, the route that everyone else seems to be taking. The route that feels better. Well I'm here to tell you today that doing the right thing will not always be easy, it won't always be fun, it won't always be what everyone else is doing... But when we do the right thing... Wow does that make God proud! I hope that when God looks down and sees me He has a smile on His face as He tells all the angels, "See there, that's my girl."

What can you do today to help someone?

Father, Please provide me with the courage and strength to do the right thing. Even if nobody else is doing it. Amen.

PY Day 2- Sugar Body Scrub

Week two is in the books! I hope you're feeling super accomplished because for the last two weeks you have been dedicated in your fellowship with God, while getting healthier. Here's a little treat for yourself for doing such a great job this week. This sugar scrub is a great way to buff off those dead skin cells we've been accumulating from sweating so much in your workouts! When rubbing the scrub into your skin it increases circulation and you'll be left with soft glowing skin when you're finished!

You'll need:
1 cup brown sugar
¼ cup melted coconut oil
1 tsp pure vanilla extract
4 drops lavender (optional)

Mix everything together, then after you've showered turn the water off and rub the sugar mixture all over your body with your hands. Once you've rubbed your whole body turn the shower back on to lukewarm water and rinse off. You'll get out of the shower feeling like a new you! I don't even put lotion on afterwards because the coconut oil is so moisturizing. You don't have to use my scrub recipe. Play around with the scent if you like and make it your own!

FYI: I try to save just a little bit and use this as a lip scrub after I've brushed my teeth for the night but I would not put it on my face.

Week Three

Meal Plan

	Breakfast	Snack 1	Lunch	Snack 2	Supper
Monday	Ham and Cheese Omelet	Peanut Butter Yogurt*	Chef Salad*	Strawberries	Tuna Salad Bowl*
Tuesday	Turmeric Oats*	Pumpkin Seeds	Tuna Salad Bowl Leftovers	Banana	Pizza*
Wednesday	Boiled Egg and Avocado Toast*	Strawberries	Pizza Leftovers	Peanut Butter Yogurt	Roasted Vegetables and Pork Chops*
Thursday	Ham and Cheese Omelet	Pumpkin Seeds	Roasted Vegetables and Pork Chops Leftovers	Banana	Turkey Taco Bowl*
Friday	Turmeric Oats	Peanut Butter Yogurt	Turkey Taco Bowl Leftovers	Srawberries	Steak and Baked Sweet Potatoes with Roasted Asparagus
Saturday	Boiled Egg and Avocado Toast	Pumpkin Seeds	Steak, Sweet Potatoes, and Asparagus Leftovers	Banana	Feta Salad*
Sunday	Willingham Tradition	Strawberries	Feta Salad Leftovers	Peanut Butter Yogurt	Eat Out

*New recipes starting on page 95

Grocery List

SPICES
HONEY
RANCH
ACV
DIJON MUSTARD
MAYONNAISE
CELERY SEED
DILL RELISH
TURMERIC
CINNAMON
GARLIC POWDER
OREGANO
RED PEPPER FLAKES
TACO SEASONING
RASPBERRY VINAIGRETTE

PRODUCE
CUCUMBER
CARROTS
LETTUCE
BELL PEPPER
STRAWBERRIES
APPLES

BANANAS
1 HEAD CAULIFLOWER
KALE CHIPS
PIZZA SAUCE
AVOCADO
1 CAN CORN
1 CAN BLACK BEANS
SWEET POTATOES
ASPARAGUS
SPINACH
SALSA
LEMONS

PROTEIN
EGGS
DELI HAM
DELI TURKEY
PEANUT BUTTER
BACON
CANS OF TUNA
WALNUTS
PEPPERONIS
1 LB. GROUND TURKEY

STEAKS
SAUSAGE
CHICKEN (GOING IN A SALAD)

DAIRY
SHREDDED CHEDDAR CHEESE
MILK
PLAIN GREEK YOGURT
SHREDDED MOZZARELLA CHEESE
GRATED PARMESAN
SOUR CREAM
FETA CHEESE CRUMBLES

GRAINS/SEEDS
CHIA SEEDS
PUMPKIN SEEDS
OATS
FLAX SEEDS
GF BREAD
RICE
GF PANCAKE MIX

Monday, Devotion 15- Shifty Sand

"The LORD is good, a strong hold in the day of trouble; and he knoweth them that trust in him."
Nahum 1:7 KJV

"The LORD is good, a strong refuge when trouble comes. He is close to those who trust in him."
Nahum 1:7 NLT Study Bible

Every year Adam and I try to go to the beach at least once. We are both drawn to the salty air, fishing, and laid back environment that the beach holds. On one of our trips Adam took me to a "secret fishing spot." We walked and walked through thick bushes, trees, and rocks. When I thought we would never get there, or a mosquito was going to take me away, the thick underbrush began to open to a beautiful white sandy beach with pine trees dotted across the water line, (yes, you read correctly… not palm trees… pine trees). While we were fishing, the whole time I was curious about those pine trees. The waves came in hard and the sands were ever changing with every wave. You could see the water line that went up the tree when high tide came in. All other trees had fallen to the mighty ocean. Yet, these simple looking pine trees held fast where they were and didn't seemed bothered by the crashing waves and shifting sand. When I mentioned the trees to Adam, he said that the trees must have a deep root system.

That's how a Christian's life is supposed to be like. God never promised we would have calm seas our whole life just because we know Him. But when the waves of life come crashing down and the sands around us (whether that be a job, loved one, finances, etc.) seem to disappear, we are to have a strong root in the word of God so that we can withstand the storm. The deeper the roots, the less you should worry about falling to the waves.

Is your root system deep in the word of God?

What's causing it to be shallow or not deep enough?

Father, I thank You for Your many blessings and for being my strong hold in the shifting sands of life, please help me deal with _________________________ so that my root system can be made even deeper. I love You, Amen.

Mondays are exciting because they are a start to a new week. If you've been slacking, forget about it and stay focused keeping your eyes on the prize. You'll have a whole new set of workouts that you haven't seen before. Complete HD #3 on page 83.

Tuesday, Devotion 16- Stand Firm

"Therefore, my beloved brethren, be ye stedfast, unmovable, always abounding in the work of the Lord, forasmuch as ye know that your labour is not in vain in the Lord." 1 Corinthians 15:58 KJV

"So, my dear brothers and sisters, be strong and immovable. Always work enthusiastically for the Lord, for you know that nothing you do for the Lord is ever useless." 1 Corinthians 15:58 NLT Study Bible

Have you ever been presented with an opportunity that sounds amazing on paper, but makes you compromise your Christian beliefs? Maybe a new job with higher pay, as long as you don't bring up God in the workplace. Maybe going to a party where the popular kids will be, but you know there will be drugs. The Bible tells us to stand firm and not to be moved. Standing up for God is not always easy and your battle between doing what God wants and what the World wants will be ever present. There are missionaries every day risking their life by standing up for God. Why? Because they understand that although standing up for Christ is not the popular thing to do here on earth, it most definitely comes with recognition from our heavenly Father.

Who are you standing up for today?

Father, In all my decisions today please let me seek Your guidance and please equip me with the strength to do what is right in Your eyes. Amen.

You worked hard yesterday and you could be sore. LD #2 on page 88 will help shape and lean out those sore muscles.

Wednesday, Devotion 17- Priceless Beauty

"Whose adorning let it not be that outward adorning of plaiting the hair, and of wearing of gold, or of putting on of apparel; But let it be the hidden man of the heart, in that which is not corruptible, even the ornament of a meek and quiet sprit, which is in the sight of God of great price." 1 Peter 3: 3-4 KJV

"Don't be concerned about the outward beauty of fancy hairstyles, expensive jewelry, or beautiful clothes. You should clothe yourselves instead with the beauty that comes from within, the unfading beauty of a gentle and quiet spirit, which is so precious to God." 1 Peter 3: 3-4 NLT Study Bible

You step on that dreaded scale and you don't see the number you're looking for. Or you caved and ate the whole chocolate cake last night. Then to make matters worse: posted everywhere are women sporting very expensive clothing that shows off their shredded midsection and long, tone legs and flawless skin with the newest hair trend that literally changed right after you cut your own hair. All those positive vibes you had about yourself vanished faster than your morning coffee.

If this sounds like you, let me remind you that although we spend hundreds if not thousands of dollars on beauty products each year, our outward beauty will be replaced with lines and wrinkles. We can't stop aging. Inward beauty however lasts a lifetime and is far more beautiful than anything we could ever wear. Yes, this is a fitness journey, but more importantly than that, this book is a spiritual journey. And if you're feeling discouraged about your weight or appearance, but have gotten closer to God. You are moving in the right direction. Keep going and don't give up.

Journal or draw how your feelings today, weather happy or sad, confident or shy. Document this journey and remind yourself that inward beauty is priceless.

Please be with me while I heal my broken self-esteem. Help me to see myself the way You see me. Let me be a light for others today. In Jesus' name, Amen.

Rest Day! You've earned it!

Thursday, Devotion 18- Where Do I Go From Here?

"Go ye therefore, and teach all nations, baptizing them in the name of the Father, and of the son, and of the Holy Ghost." Matthew 28: 19 KJV

"Therefore, go and make disciples of all the nations, baptizing them in the name of the Father and the Son and the Holy Spirit." Matthew 28:19 NLT Study Bible

God doesn't categorize us into groups by height, weight, gender, or color. He knows everything about each of us specifically and our walk with Him is as individualized as your fingerprint. Although your walk is different from anyone else, the journey to get there is the same format for everyone.

First of all, know that once you become a Christian your sins are forgiven through the blood of Jesus Christ. You are then filled with the Holy Spirit which gives you this desire to please God. How do you live a life for God?

We should **pray** daily and often, talk to Him. He already knows what's in your heart but He longs to hear it from you. He's the friend that will never tell your secrets or belittle your worries.

Fellowship with other Christians. Find a mentor, join a church, and surround yourself with positive Christian people that will help build you up and encourage you when life gets hard.

Read your Bible and study God's word. The more we understand and learn about the Bible the less likely the devil can come in and tear us down.

Christ also tells us to **share** the gospel with everyone we come in contact with. Witness to those around you. How? If you are a Christian God has blessed you with a testimony. You may not know every verse of the Bible but you do know what our great God has done for you. Share it.

Sharing the gospel segues into **doing** good works. The Bible tells us in Ephesians 2:8 that it is not by works that we are saved but by faith. It is with this faith that we long to do good works and please God.

To recap we should Pray, Fellowship, Read, Share, and Do.

Are you where you need to be today?

Father, You have equipped me with a marvelous gift, You have given me a testimony which I now know I should openly share with others. Please let doors be opened for me to have a chance to share my testimony with someone today. Thank You God for all You do.

If you haven't already noticed, you have more workouts this week than previously. It will get harder, but the hope is that you're getting stronger. Your workout for today is HD #4 on page 84.

Friday, Devotion 19- Put Me in Coach

"Wherefore, my beloved, as ye have always obeyed, not as in my presence only, but now much more in my absence, work out your own salvation with fear and trembling." Philippians 2: 12 KJV

"Dear friends, you always followed my instructions when I was with you. And now that I am away, it is even more important. Work hard to show the results of your salvation, obeying God with deep reverence and fear." Philippians 2:12 NLT Study Bible

Hypothetically speaking, let's say you coach a baseball team. It's the World Series! Bottom of the ninth, bases are loaded, you're down by one and the other team's power hitter is up to bat that has already hit it out of the park once during this game… You have a choice. You can put on the mound your best pitcher that practices every day and has a good rapport with your catcher and the team. OR you can put in the guy that never shows up to practice, doesn't listen to the catcher when he's giving signals, and is not a team player. The answer seems obvious, doesn't it?

So now let's look at this scenario in a way that conveys our own life. Sometimes we see really bad things happening to Christians. Maybe some bad things have happened in your own life. Then we turn around and see some really bad people we know aren't Christians seeming to have everything figured out in life with nothing bad ever seeming to come their way. Why does God let this happen? This world is the only hope sinners have at having a good life. Because after this life they will spend an eternity in Hell. But for the Christian, we have hope after this life. We have Jesus Christ! So next time something bad is happening in your life, take pride in the difficult times. Because God thinks you can handle the bottom of the ninth pressure and come out victorious. After all, what coach would send out the worst player to finish out such an important game?

Turn in your Bibles and read Philippians 2: 12-18.

Father, You must really have faith in me because You know what's been going on in my life and you know that I am overwhelmed with _______________, but I thank You! I thank You and praise Your name because if it wasn't for You there is no way I could make it in the life. Help me to hold my head high and remember that You are always there when life gets me down. Amen.

LD #3 on page 89.

Saturday, Devotion 20- New Car Smell

"What? Know ye not that your body is the temple of the Holy Ghost which is in you, which ye have of God, and ye are not your own? For ye are bought with a price: therefore glorify God in your body, and in your spirit, which are God's." 1 Corinthians 6: 19-20 KJV

"Don't you realize that your body is the temple of the Holy Spirit, who lives in you and was given to you by God? You do not belong to yourself, for God bought you with a high price. So you must honor God with your body." 1 Corinthians 6:19-20 NLT Study Bible

I remember when I purchased my first car. I had worked for several years doing odd jobs and raising and selling bottle calves until I was finally able to afford an early 90s model Toyota Corolla. The back window wouldn't raise, there were stains and tears in the seat, dents on the exterior, and it didn't have a CD player (which was a big deal back in high school). Yes, one might've called my first car a "junker". But I didn't care!

I vacuumed it out, put a pina colada scented tree and lei on the rearview mirror, purchased a foam steering wheel cover, and installed a CD player. Lola was her name and she was perfect despite her flaws. She got me from point A to point B and in return I took such good care of her. I would wash her, wouldn't let anyone eat in her, I would have the oil changed, brakes checked, and tires rotated regularly. Why is it that we take so much pride in our material possessions and let our bodies and our health be pushed to the backburner?

Despite our flaws we are perfect in God's eyes. He loves us and made us in His own image so we should take care of ourselves.

Is there something you are doing, or not doing, today that you know is effecting your body and health?

Father, Help me to remember that my body is a temple. Not just any temple, a temple that houses the Holy Spirit. A temple that is not my own. Please let me remember that when it comes to taking care of my body. Amen.

Fitness Dare Day!
You know the routine. Go to page 91 and pick out which fun FD you're going to do today!
Make it fun and make it count!

Sunday, Devotion 21- Getting More ZZZ

"Come unto me, all ye that labour and are heavy laden, and I will give you rest." Matthew 11:28 KJV

"Then Jesus said, "Come to me, all of you who are weary and carry heavy burdens, and I will give you rest." Matthew 11:28 NLT Study Bible

Rest is mentioned a lot in the Bible and dates back as early as the creation of the world. If it's mentioned a great deal, it must be important. If you look up the definition of rest you'll find words such as "inactivity, a brief pause, peace of mind or spirit, freedom from activity." When God rested on the seventh day of creation it wasn't because He was tired or even because He needed a rest. I personally feel like He did this as an example for what we should do.

Our bodies can only go so long physically without rest. Our metabolism and health both suffer if we do not get enough sleep. We also need to rest mentally, a chance to re-charge the batteries and step back from what's going on in our lives causing us stress. Spiritually, the Bible tells us to lay down our heavy burdens and God our Father will give us rest. Rest in all aspects of life is important. And it is with this rest that we can slow down and give God the praise and glory He rightfully deserves.

Try to go to bed at least 30 minutes earlier than you typically would all next week. Also try tonight when you're doing your PY session to unplug from all electronics and let your mind rest.

If there is something causing you to not sleep at night, no matter how big or small, lay it before God and receive that peace of mind you've been longing for.

Father, I am burdened with _____________________. It keeps me up at night and I'm tired of my mind racing in circles. I lay this burden at Your feet and humbly ask that you take it from me and bring about a peace of mind. Forgive me for not bringing this to You sooner. Thank You for always loving me. Amen.

PY Day #3

Today's pamper session is geared toward your pearly whites and oral hygiene. Oil pulling is an ancient method of ridding the mouth of toxins and bacteria using coconut oil. Your mouth is well… disgusting! And I love coconut oil for its anti-bacterial and anti-fungal properties.

All you need is 1tbl of coconut oil and 20 minutes. Yes, this seems like a very long time (and I'm going to be honest, I get super board when I do this so I try reading a book or going ahead and taking my shower to pass the time). Simply put the coconut oil in your mouth and swish around like mouthwash for 20 minutes. Try not to swallow it, spit it out and brush your teeth as normal. If you don't feel comfortable doing this then pick something else that you can do to pamper your body for a few minutes before bed.

NOTE: When I feel a sore throat coming on or I'm already sick I will do this every day for about a week to help combat the sickness.

Week Four

Meal Plan

	Breakfast	Snack 1	Lunch	Snack 2	Supper
Monday	Eggs, B-B Muffins* and Sausage	Apple	Chef Salad*	Carrots and Hummus	Stuffed Peppers*
Tuesday	Clean Pancakes*	Nut Mix*	Stuffed Peppers Leftovers	Fruit	BBQ with Broccoli Slaw*
Wednesday	Chocolate Smoothie*	Apple	BBQ Leftovers	Carrots and Hummus	Chicken Caesar Salad*
Thursday	Eggs, B-B Muffins and Sausage	Nut Mix	Chicken Caesar Salad Leftovers	Fruit	Turkey Chili*
Friday	Clean Pancakes	Apple	Turkey Chili Leftovers	Carrots and Hummus	Salmon Broccoli and Rice
Saturday	Chocolate Smoothie	Nut Mix	Salmon Broccoli and Rice Leftovers	Fruit	Chicken and Vegetables*
Sunday	Willingham Tradition	Apple	Chicken and Vegetables Leftovers	Carrots and Hummus	Eat Out

*Recipes in the back

Grocery List

SPICES
HONEY
COCONUT OIL
CINNAMON
VANILLA
BAKING POWDER
BAKING SODA
SEA SALT
PEPPER
SYRUP
DARK CHOCOLATE CHIPS
CELERY SEED
GROUND MUSTARD
DRIED BAY LEAF
LIQUID STEAK SEASONING
WORCESTERSHIRE SAUCE
ACV
MAYONNAISE
BBQ SAUCE
CACAO POWDER
CAESAR DRESSING
FRESH PARSLEY
CHILI POWDER
CUMIN POWDER
PAPRIKA
TURMERIC
FRESH ROSEMARY

PRODUCE
BANANAS (6 AT LEAST)
APPLE SAUCE
BLUEBERRIES
APPLES
CARROTS
SPINACH
ICEBERG LETTUCE
BELL PEPPERS (4)
CAN OF DICED TOMATOES
AND PEPPERS
TOMATO JUICE
DRIED CRANBERRIES
FRUIT OF CHOICE (FOR
SNACKS)
ONIONS (2)
BAG OF BROCCOLI SLAW
LEMONS
ZUCCHINI
FROZEN STRAWBERRIES
ROMAINE LETTUCE
GARLIC
SMALL CAN TOMATO PASTE
CAN OF TOMATO SAUCE
FROZEN BROCCOLI
VEGETABLES OF CHOICE
(FOR
SUPPER SATURDAY)

PROTEIN
EGGS
SAUSAGE
HUMMUS
CUBED HAM
CUBED TURKEY
BACON
12 OZ. ITALIAN SAUSAGE
1-2LB DEER ROAST
NUT BUTTER
CHICKEN BREAST
1 LB. GROUND TURKEY
CAN CHILI BEANS
CAN KIDNEY BEANS
SALMON FILLETS
ALMOND MILK

DAIRY
CHEDDAR CHEESE (2 BAGS)
BUTTER
PARMESAN CHEESE
MILK

GRAINS/SEEDS
WALNUTS
GF FLOUR
BROWN RICE
GROUND FLAX SEED
ALMONDS
OLD FASHION OATS
CHIA SEEDS
GF PANCAKE MIX

Monday, Devotion 22- Let it Go

"Wherefore, my beloved brethren, let every man be swift to hear, slow to speak, slow to wrath: For the wrath of man worketh not the righteousness of God." KJV

"Understand this, my dear brothers and sisters: You must all be quick to listen, slow to speak, and slow to get angry. Human anger does not produce the righteousness God desires." NLT Study Bible

Anger is like a weed. At first it starts out small, but if not pulled up and dealt with it can easily take over your garden and smother your flowers. The Bible tells us to be slow to anger and quick to listen. This can be very hard when the devil is telling you that you deserve to be angry and you should hold a grudge, or you have the right to give that person a piece or your mind because you are in the right. Where all those things might be true, it still doesn't justify in the Lord's eyes to be angry with a fellow brother or sister.

The devil would love nothing more than for us to always be angry at one another, because if we are angry with our fellow man we are not sharing the gospel with them. If we are angry and fly off the handle, unbelievers will look at that and think, "That Christian is no better than myself so why should I go to church, or change my ways?" Anger can harden your soul and steal your joy, which is exactly what the devil wants.

Don't let the devil win today. If you are angry about a past transgression with a fellow man, pull that weed up and throw it out of your garden. Talk to that person and make things right, which is pleasing to the Lord. Be slow to anger and quick to listen. Just because we don't agree with someone doesn't mean we have to take our wrath out on them. It's amazing at how much better you feel when that hate and anger towards another person dissipates and you give it to God.

Don't let the weeds of anger and sin smother your joy.

Are you angry with someone today? Let it go, give it to God and move on with your life.

Father, Provide me with the strength to let go of past transgressions. I want to thank You so much for allowing me to be forgiven of my sins and never holding a grudge about me even though I know I deserve it. Amen.

Your workout for today is HD #3 on page 89.

Tuesday, Devotion 23- Master

"He that loveth silver shall not be satisfied with silver; nor he that loveth abundance with increase: this [is] also vanity." Ecclesiastes 5: 10 KJV

"Those who love money will never have enough. How meaningless to think that wealth brings true happiness!" Ecclesiastes 5: 10 NLT Study Bible

Bills, cars, clothes, groceries, phones, luxuries, houses, jewelry, fuel, school supplies… do you know what all of these things have in common? They cost money. Society would love us to think that if you're not on top of the latest trend or if you don't have the newest gadget out then you're not going to be happ, but that way of thinking leads to debt.

Debt only makes you crave more money, because you're trying to get out of debt, so that you can buy more stuff. You begin to only think about things in the way of dollar signs. Be very careful about doing this. The Bible tells us that you can't serve two masters, you either choose to serve God or money. When you choose to serve money you become more and more in debt. To pay off that debt you work more, taking time away from your family and the Lord. When even working overtime is not enough to pay your bills, you start to worry. That worry leads to resentment, which leads you on a downward spiral and away from God.

But when you serve our Lord, you realize that you need to stop the spending. Work towards paying off the debt you've already accumulated so that you can focus more on doing God's will. And you learn to be happy in the situation you're in and be thankful for what you already have.

Who is your master today?

A good way to start working towards paying off your debt is to write out all of your expenses on a piece of paper and divide it into two columns. The first column is bills that you will always have (like utilities, tithe, and insurance). In the second column write down your debt i.e. car payment, hospital bills, house payment, boat payment etc. starting with the least amount owed to the highest amount owed.

Add up what you make in a month and what both columns add up to then see what you have left each month after paying all the bills.

Column 1 + Column 2 – Monthly pay = money left

Next make a budget. With the remaining money you have after bills, put that money into three different groups, gas/groceries, emergency fund, and debt reduction. Each month take out a certain amount for gas/groceries. Then put your desired amount into your emergency fund for those "didn't expect my car to break down" moments and then everything else goes towards paying off whatever is listed on the top of column two.

LD #2 on page 88 is your workout of the day.

Wednesday, Devotion 24- You're Getting Warmer

"For our God is a consuming fire." Hebrews 12:29 KJV

"For our God is a devouring fire." Hebrews 12:29 NLT Study Bible

     If you had to pick, what type of Christian would you be? To me there are three different classifications of a Christian. You have the Cold Christian; this person has been saved, therefore they will go to heaven thanks to God's gift of eternal salvation (John 10:23). But they have done nothing in their life to show gratitude towards our heavenly Father and others can't see a difference in them. They do the same things they did before God was in their life without change.

     You then have the lukewarm Christian, this person was on fire for God at one point in their life, but for whatever reason they have slowed down. They are not active in their church and people can't see a difference in their lives anymore. What was once right and wrong, black and white, has now formed a gray area in their lives and they don't stand out for Christ. If this is you and you think it's because God has dealt in your life and you fulfilled your purpose so now you can just live and be comfortable in your routine, let me say that if you are still breathing, God has a plan for you and a job to do. He doesn't want your light to be hidden under a rock but to shine for Him on the mountain for all to see.

     Then there is the Fiery Christian. This person is on fire for God and those around them notice how something about them is different than others. They strive daily to do the will of God and to help others find that eternal salvation that they have. They spread the gospel night and day and with all things bring glory to God.

     I wish I could say that I was a fiery Christian all the time, but I'm not. However, my goal is to always strive to be on fire for God more than I was the day before.

So... which one are you? Which one do you want to be? And what are you going to do about it to get there?

That once roaring fire is now but a flame. Please come into my life and renew that fire I once had. Help me to read Your words daily so that I can receive a blessing and thus bless someone else. In Jesus' name, Amen.

Today is a rest day. Focus on resting up your body and putting good food into it to help you recover from the workouts on Monday and Tuesday.

Thursday, Devotion 25- To Work or Not to Work?

"The soul of the sluggard desireth, and [hath] nothing: but the soul of the diligent shall be made fat." Proverbs 13:4 KJV

"Lazy people want much but get little, but those who work hard will prosper." Proverbs 13:4 NLT Study Bible

Wouldn't it be troubling if a surgeon decided to be lazy that day and not be diligent during an operation? Or what if the crew working on fixing the red light in town decided to be lazy and not work today? The laziness of these individuals could turn into multiple people getting hurt. What if it was something that didn't seem so horrible and you just skipped your homework for that day? Or just didn't do the laundry? The Bible warns about being lazy and not doing the work that needs to be done. It doesn't matter what the Lord has laid at our feet for the day, whether it be homework or a lifesaving surgery. We are to work hard and give it our all and in doing so we will glorify the Lord and prosper. The same can be said for your daily workouts, give it your all and you will see results!!!

To help combat laziness write out a To Do list for the day and plan time in-between activities to rest and relax for a few moments before beginning the next activity. Marking things off your list will help you feel accomplished and motivated to keep going!

To Do List

1.   6.
2.   7.
3.   8.
4.   9.
5.   10.

Father, No matter how big or small the task, help me to be glad in it and give the work You've prepared for the day one hundred percent. Amen.

Get ready and excited to burn fat while feeling good about yourself for taking time to get your workout on. You have done so great! Don't give up! Remember that you can modify all exercises to fit your individual needs. Make it easier or harder but do the workout! HD #4 page 84.

Friday, Devotion 26- Finding Joy

"And God shall wipe away all tears from their eyes: and there shall be no more death, neither sorrow, nor crying, neither shall there be any more pain; for the former things are passed away." Revelation 21:4 KJV

"He will wipe every tear from their eyes, and there will be no more death or sorrow or crying or pain. All these things are gone forever." Revelation 21:4 NLT Study Bible

We've all had those really bad days where nothing went right. Sometimes those bad days make us feel like we have a bad life. This is the smoke and mirrors the devil wants to put in front of your face to rid you of your joy. Those that are not walking in Christ would get discouraged and try to feel that joyless void with worldly pleasures. Whether that be going on a shopping spree, recreational drugs, binge eating, or sexual immorality: all those things may make you feel good in the moment, but they never last and it leaves you searching for another way to find a temporary joy.

Let me share with you a joy that abounds all others, a joy that will be forever present as long as your eyes are towards God. If you are a Christian you should have this type of joy that I'm referring to. The joy of knowing that no matter what bad things happen here on the earth, no matter the hurt, or the pain: you are going to be with our Lord Jesus Christ forever and ever! The lame will walk! The blind will see! Every tear will be wiped away and there will be no more sorrow but forever shouting and singing of praise to our great and mighty God.

For you see, the pleasures of this life are temporary and will not bring everlasting joy. When those bad days inevitably come, look to God for your joy and remember waiting for us in heaven is God's outstretched arms in the most beautiful place you have ever seen with our loved ones that have went on before us. Wow! How wonderful and amazing!

Want to learn more about heaven? Look up these other verses:
Revelation 21
John 14: 1-3
Philippians 3:20-21
Luke 23:43

Lord God, I find myself looking to the world for joy instead of looking towards You. Please help me, and those I know to stop looking for temporary joy and instead look
towards the actual Creator of Joy. Although I know very little about heaven, I know You will be there. Thank You so much for that! Amen.

Do workout LD #3 on page 89.

Saturday, Devotion 27- Powerful Prayer

"And this is the confidence that we have in Him, that, if we ask any thing according to His will, He heareth us." 1 John 5:14 KJV

"And we are confident that He hears us whenever we ask for anything that pleases Him." 1 John 5:14 NLT Study Bible

When I was in the hospital having my second child my parents had to watch my first born because he wasn't allowed to stay in the hospital. I knew he was okay, but I still wanted my parents to call me so I could check on him and hear his sweet little voice. I know that when my babies get bigger and head to school (and I get past ugly crying when I drop them off), I will still want them to tell me about their day. Even if I already know what happened because I want them to be the ones that tell me, not their teachers.

This is exactly how God feels about us. He already knows absolutely everything that has went on in our day, good and bad, but He wants us to be the ones to tell Him. Prayer is much more special than a few words before meals or at bedtime. But it should be a constant conversation with our Lord. There's no special words or phrases you need to say, no special place you need to be, and no special time of day. You can talk to God anytime about anything anywhere. This is confirmed in the Word when it says that as long as our prayers are in the will of God He will hear us.

When we pray we should give God praise and thanksgiving for all His blessings, confess our sins, ask for help to not repeat the same mistakes, and then pour our hearts out to God and tell Him what's on your mind. He also wants us to pray for our fellow man. Prayer is powerful and God is waiting to hear from you today.

Father, Your warm embrace comforts me in my time of need. You are an amazing artist because this world You've made is beautiful. Forgive me where I've failed you and disappointed You. Help me to learn from my mistakes and run from the devil. Please help all those that need Your love and support. Help me make it a habit to pray daily and often. Amen.

Another Saturday is here and it's time for you to pick out what FD you're going to be doing today. Make sure you've picked out a dare you haven't completed yet and go have fun. You can find the FD on page 91.

Sunday, Devotion 28-That Book With Its Cover

"Judge not according to the appearance, but judge righteous judgement." John 7: 24 KJV

"Look beneath the surface so you can judge correctly." John 7:24 NLT Study Bible

A few years back I went with my husband to his company picnic. It was a family gathering so everyone brought their children. Everyone was dressed formally except one teenage boy. He was in dirty clothing, had holes in his shirt, too skinny for his frame, and I couldn't help but notice body odor when he walked past. He didn't appear to have any family there so I assumed it was a new hire from the temp service my husband's company uses. In my head, I was already thinking "he's probably made some wrong choices in his life and that's why he looks like that, possibly drugs."

SHAME. ON. ME.

Come to find out this boy had seen more in his short life than I could have ever dreamed of. He had watched his mother die, his father was in prison, and was left to basically raise himself. How quickly we are to judge someone else because of their appearances. Here was a boy that was lost, heartbroken, and I'm sure scared. Yet he was putting on the bravest face he could muster. I consider myself a professional people watcher, and he knew his clothes were not like everyone else and that he looked out of place. But he came anyway, despite the fact that I'm sure more than just me were judging him. And no, I never said anything about the boy out loud, but thinking it is just as bad. The Bible tells us to not judge others based on appearance, but righteous judgement, meaning what's on the inside. It also tells us to not judge others unless we ourselves want to be judged (Luke 6:37). So next time you look someone up and down and begin to judge them remember that there is always more than meets the eye.

Father, Please forgive me for being so superficial and so quick to judge others before getting to know them. Help me to instead of being judgmental, to think about what they may be going through and love them the way You do. Amen.

Today we are going to pamper your face! Weather you have dry skin, acne prone skin, or oily skin this all around two ingredient face mask is affordable, easy, effective, and the ingredients are found in your kitchen!

You'll need: ½ tsp turmeric and 2 tbsp. honey. That's it! Just mix in a bowl and then smooth over your face. Let set for at least 20 minutes then wash off. The turmeric will improve the integrity of your skin and fight breakouts while the honey will help hydrate and clear your skin. I love just lying on the couch and chilling out for a few minutes because be warned! The honey begins to start melting on your face and if you're walking around everywhere it could drip off the face and make a mess.

Enjoy clear beautiful skin while praising our Lord and preparing for the upcoming work week.

Week Five

Meal Plan

	Breakfast	Snack 1	Lunch	Snack 2	Supper
Monday	Loaded Omelet*	Blueberries and Walnuts	Chef Salad*	Cheese Stick	Turkey Taco Bowl*
Tuesday	Turmeric Oats*	Edamame	Turkey Taco Bowl Leftovers	Orange	Chef Salad
Wednesday	Eggs and B-B Muffins*	Blueberries and Walnuts	Chef Salad Leftovers	Cheese stick	Shrimp Scampi Pasta*
Thursday	Loaded Omelet	Edamame	Shrimp Scampi Pasta Leftovers	Orange	Very Veggie Spaghetti*
Friday	Turmeric Oats	Cheese Stick	Very Veggie Spaghetti Leftovers	Blueberries and Walnuts	Pizza*
Saturday	Eggs and B-B Muffins	Edamame	Pizza Leftovers	Orange	Steak with Sweet Potatoes and Asparagus
Sunday	Willingham Tradition	Blueberries and Walnuts	Steak with Sweet Potatoes and Asparagus Leftovers	Cheese Stick	Eat Out

*Recipes in the back starting on page 95

Grocery List

SPICES
COCONUT OIL
RANCH DRESSING
TACO SEASONING
HONEY
TURMERIC
CINNAMON
VANILLA EXTRACT
BAKING POWDER
BAKING SODA
SEA SALT
PEPPER
ACV
CHICKEN STOCK
RED PEPPER FLAKES
GARLIC POWDER
DRIED OREGANO

PRODUCE
MUSHROOMS
BELL PEPPERS (2)
SPINACH
BLUEBERRIES
ICEBERG LETTUCE

CARROTS
1 CAN BLACK BEANS
1 CAN CORN
EDAMAME
ORANGES
BANANAS
APPLESAUCE
FROZEN BROCCOLI
GARLIC
LEMONS
16OZ SPAGHETTI SAUCE
ONION
1 CAULIFLOWER HEAD
KALE CHIPS
PIZZA SAUCE
SWEET POTATOES
ASPARAGUS

PROTEIN
DELI HAM
DELI TURKEY
BACON
1 LB. GROUND BEEF
1 LB. GROUND TURKEY
NUT BUTTER

BAG OF FROZEN SHRIMP
PEPPERONI
STEAKS

DAIRY
SHREDDED CHEDDAR
CHEESE
MILK
CHEESE STICKS
GRATED PARMESAN CHEESE
GRATED ROMANO CHEESE
SHREDDED MOZZARELLA
CHEESE
BUTTER

GRAINS/SEEDS
RICE
OATS
FLAX SEEDS
GF FLOUR
GF SPAGHETTI NOODLES
GF PASTA
GF PANCAKE MIX
***CHEESE CLOTH (IF
YOU'RE MAKING HOME-
MADE PIZZA CRUST)

Monday, Devotion 29- Forgiveness

"Then said Jesus, "Father, forgive them; for they know not what they do." And they parted his raiments and cast lots." Luke 23:34 KJV

"Jesus said, "Father, forgive them, for they don't know what they are doing." And the soldiers gambled for his clothes by throwing dice. Luke 23:34 NLT Study Bible

I love getting some time to play with the kids in their bedroom. However, it never ceases to amaze me that in their sea of toys, they both want to play with that one toy the other has. Even though Avery is a good bit smaller than her big brother she can hold her own pretty well in the battle of the toys. In those instances where she doesn't get her way, she gets so mad at Reed and will begin to throw a huge fit! Momma has to step in and make Reed apologize or give Avery a different toy to play with. It's mind blowing how hard she screamed and pitched a fit, then just like turning off a light switch, she's back to her loving self, playing with her big brother and having a good time. Wouldn't it be great if we could all be that way when it came to forgiveness?

Some would say, "My situation is a lot worse than a toy being stolen, you don't know what they've done to me." You may be right, your situation could be worse, but aren't you glad God doesn't give US what WE deserve by holding back forgiveness which is an eternity in Hell separated from Him? Matthew 6:15 tells us that as long as we forgive others God will also forgive us.

Is your situation worse than being beat to an inch of your life and then hung on a cross where you were tortured until your death? And yet, even while going through more pain and suffering than we can comprehend Jesus still said, "Father forgive them." I don't know about you, but I know of nothing someone has done to me worse that what Jesus endured.

Are you holding back forgiveness today? Why?

Are you seeking forgiveness from someone else?

Father, Thank You so much for sending you son Jesus Christ to suffer and die on the cross for my sins. I see now that if Jesus can forgive His murderers (and me) then I need to forgive _______________________. Please help me to forgive them and move on with my life. Father, I lay this at Your feet and I don't want to take it up as my burden anymore. I also pray that You forgive me for _______________________ . You know my heart, and for that I am thankful. In Your name I pray, Amen.

HD #5 on page 85 is your workout for today!

Tuesday, Devotion 30- Good Medicine

"A merry heart doeth good like a medicine: but a broken spirit drieth the bones." Proverbs 17:22 KJV

"A cheerful heart is good medicine, but a broken spirit saps a person's strength." Proverbs 17:22 NLT Study Bible

I have always heard that it takes more muscles to frown than it does to smile. I have also heard that if you keep thinking positively your brain and body will start to believe it. I believe both of the above statements to be true. Why? Because it tells us in scripture that laughter and positive thinking are both good medicine.

We already know that every good gift comes from our Heavenly Father (James 1:17). So we can firmly believe that God created laughter, fun, happiness, joy, and love. In the world we live in today, there are so many stumbling blocks that obstruct our path which cause us to think poorly of ourselves and others. We get discouraged and begin to have a bad attitude, and the wrong outlook on life can quickly take over like a cloud covering the sun. I challenge you today that when times get hard and all seems hopeless, remember that a merry heart is good medicine for the soul. Remember who your Heavenly Father is and what He's done for you. Remember to smile… it's contagious.

Precious Heavenly Father, I thank You so much for creating laughter, love, and joy. You give us these gifts so we can continue this walk of life even when times seem hard, lonely, or just unbearable. You know what's on my mind so I really need help today to remember to smile and be positive because ______________________________ is going on in my life. Help me to remember that You don't want me to be discouraged, but encouraged, so that I can be a good example for others watching me. Amen.

LD #4 on page 90 is today's workout. Go smash it out and get sweaty and smile while doing it because you're getting healthier which equals happier!

Wednesday, Devotion 31- Love Doesn't Mean Acceptance

"But I say unto you, love your enemies, bless them that curse you, do good to them that hate you, and pray for them which despitefully use you, and persecute you." Matthew 5: 44 KJV

"But I say, love your enemies! Pray for those who persecute you!" Matthew 5: 44 NLT Study Bible

My husband and I have been married for going on eight years. It has been hard and not all days have been the best days. But when asked how we have kept our marriage alive and thriving I tell people that it takes hard work, communication, putting God first, then putting your spouse next, and praying for them (just to name a few). All of these things are under an umbrella of love.

Did you know we are commanded to love and pray for everyone, even our enemies? Now this commandment that the Lord gives us can sometimes be twisted around to make us feel better about what we're doing in our lives. That God is okay with everything we do, even if it's in sin, because He loves us. So let me clear up some things; God commanded us to love our enemies, He never said that we had to agree with them (notice I never said hate, but agree). If someone is doing something that is biblically wrong, yes we should disagree and not be involved in that sin, but we are to love them and pray for them just as we would our spouse or best friend. We as Christians can disagree with what someone is doing, (just like how you and your spouse or best friend disagree sometimes), but at the end of the day we still love them.

If someone is doing something that is biblically wrong, we as Christians can disagree with what they are doing. Don't misconstrue the concept of love for acceptance. We as Christians can stand firm in our beliefs and refuse to go down a path of acceptance of all things despite what today's world would like us to think. The world [devil] tells us to accept, but Christ tells us to love.

Lord, Loving my enemies is so very hard. And in today's world you know people would like for me to think I'm in the wrong for disagreeing with things that I know are scripturally wrong in Your eyes. They make it seem like if I don't accept the "norms" of today's world then I'm a bad person, but please give me the strength to stand up for what I know is right and help me to love those that persecute me and pray for them regardless of how they view me. In that same way I pray for my spouse ______________, help them to have a great day, a safe day, and most importantly a day that honors You. Help me to make a commitment to love everyone today. I can only do this if You help me. Thank You for always being there for me. In Jesus' name, Amen.

HD #6 on page 86 is the workout for today! Don't make excuses, you've got this! Don't quit!

Thursday, Devotion 32- Gratitude List

"These things I have spoken unto you, that in me ye might have peace. In the world ye shall have tribulation: but be of good cheer; I have overcome the world." John 16:33 KJV

"I have told you all this so that you may have peace in me. Here on earth you will have many trials and sorrows. But take heart, because I have overcome the world." John 16:33 NLT Study Bible

Are you a "glass half empty" or "glass half full" type of person? Life will get us down, and eventually everything in the world, including the people around you, will disappoint you. Your car is having trouble, your relationships are broken, your health is declining, someone you love has hurt you, you're financially struggling, and you hate your job… I could take this whole page to write all the negativity that will eventually come around in your life. But when you read the Bible it tells us to be of good cheer because our Heavenly Father is bigger than any problem we will face here on earth. We are too look at life in a "glass half full" perspective. So instead of making a mental list of all the bad things that are going wrong for the day, take a little extra time in the given space to write out a gratitude list. Write down all those things we take for granted on a daily basis and give thanks to our Lord for overcoming the world.

_________________ _________________ _________________

_________________ _________________ _________________

_________________ _________________ _________________

_________________ _________________ _________________

Dear Lord, Thank You for overcoming the world. I'm sorry that I so quickly forget all the wonderful blessings you bestow on me daily. Help me to look at life in a "glass half full" perspective and hopefully in doing so, shine some light in someone else's day. I love you! Amen.

Remember when I told you that the goal of this book was to help you become your own body's advocate? Well today is going to be a test. It is a YC day! That means that you choose what you want to do today. It can be any workout from this book or go make up your own. Just make sure your listening to your body. I challenge you to get in a good sweat today! If you work out today, then you pass this test!

Friday, Devotion 33- Leap of Faith

"Fear thou not; for I am with thee: be not dismayed; for I am thy God: I will strengthen thee; yea, I will help thee; yea, I will uphold thee with the right hand of my righteousness." Isaiah 41:10 KJV

"Don't be afraid, for I am with you. Don't be discouraged, for I am your God. I will strengthen you and help you. I will hold you up with my victorious right hand." Isaiah 41:10 NLT Study Bible

In high school during the summer I worked as a lifeguard and taught swim lessons. One little girl I taught in particular would cling to her momma for dear life! Only glancing at the water over her beach towel with fear and dreaded anticipation. You could tell she wanted to jump in like all the other kids, but felt safer wrapped in her beach towel. It took me telling her that I was going to hold both of her hands and I would not let go before she ever took that jump into the pool. I never let go of her hands, and when she came up out of the water she had a look of victory! She quickly swam to the stairs, got out, and came back over to jump again. When I asked if she needed my hands again she said, "No, I know you'll be right there to get me if I don't come up."

Sometimes we get comfy in life, we settle into a routine and feel safe in our little bubble we've made for ourselves and think, "Yep I've got this life thing whipped." Then God asks you to get out of that bubble and do something you're not comfortable doing. If you're experiencing a situation like that in your own life then know that taking that leap of faith in Christ is better than being out of His will and being "comfy". Scripture tells us that God's got you in His hands and He'll never let go. We should take that leap of faith and do God's will because He will always be there ready to pull us up from the water.

Father, It's amazing how you created the world; every animal, tree, plant, ray of sunshine. Every spark of laughter and love comes from You. I too quickly forget this when You ask me to go out on a limb and have faith. I know You love me and I know You will also watch over me. Please let Your will be done in my life and help me to take that leap of faith now, or be ready to do so in the future. Thank You again for all your great blessings.
Amen.

HD #1 is your workout for the day! You'll find it on page 81.

Saturday, Devotion 34- Thirsty

"Jesus answered and said unto her, 'If thou knewest the gift of God, and who it is that saith to thee, Give me to drink; thou wouldest have asked of him, and he would have given thee living water.'" John 4:10 KJV

"Jesus replied, 'If you only knew the gift God has for you and who you are speaking to, you would ask me, and I would give you living water.'" John 4:10 NLT Study Bible

Jesus tells the woman mentioned in the scripture about a thirst quenching water that would change her life if she only drinks from it. Jesus was of course talking about His gift of eternal salvation, however there is another type of thirst we as Christians should have: a thirst for knowledge, understanding, comfort, etc. This thirst can only be quenched if we dive into the Word of God, read our Bible, and go to our Lord daily in fellowship and prayer. Unlike the living water Jesus speaks about, if we stop drinking water our physical self-suffers. The same can be said about our spiritual self. If we don't water our souls they will suffer and eventually die.

Are you watering your life today?

Read John 4:1-26 to find out what happened with the woman and the living water.

Lord, Thank You so much for sending Jesus to die on the cross for my sins so that I could have the living water that scripture talks about. Help me to water my soul daily and be a Christian example for those around me. In Jesus' name, Amen.

FD day!!! Go to page 91 and pick a FD that you have not attempted yet and go have a blast while burning some calories in the process.

Sunday, Devotion 35- Run From Sin and Sugar

"This I say then, walk in the Spirit, and ye shall not fulfil the lust of the flesh." Galatians 5:16 KJV

"So I say, let the Holy Spirit guide your lives. Then you won't be doing what your sinful nature craves." Galatians 5:16 NLT Study Bible

We all know I have a love hate relationship with sugar. I used to love consuming sugary foods, but I knew they were doing really bad things to my body. The more sugar I ingested the more sugar my body craved. When I decided to cut back on refined sugars it was not easy. The first week I found myself literally day dreaming about a gooey brownie or a huge piece of key lime pie. I had horrible withdrawal headaches and I didn't think it was ever going to end. Finally, a week passed and the headaches subsided, but the day-dreaming didn't. I found other dessert alternatives that were not packed with refined sugars and another week came and went. Before I knew it, I had almost completely cut refined sugars out of my diet and was actually craving healthier snack options. I was able to have portion control and I didn't see the enticement of the gooey brownie I once craved.

Although there are more addictions much more serious than sugar, to break the cycle of sin is the same concept of breaking away from sugar. When there is sin in our lives the Holy Spirit lets us know that what we're doing is wrong. But it is sometimes really hard to break away from that sin, because just like sugar, your body craves it and you are consumed in that sin. Once you make that decision to break away from the sin you're going to need the Lord to help you get through it because the devil will try any way he can to get you to stay in your sinful nature. You could potentially lose friends, relationships, and family members by leaving your life of sin. It will be very hard in the beginning, but as long as you're walking with God you will get past it. And finally, you'll be able to look back and see the sin and relationships that once consumed your life and think, "What did I ever see in that?"

Whether its sugar, your appearances, drugs, a toxic relationship, shopping, etc. if your day is consumed with those things and you're putting them ahead of your Heavenly Father, it is a sin.

What sins are you holding onto today?

Lord, Your love for me is unbelievable. My punishment for my sins should be death and eternal separation from You in Hell, but You love me enough to heal me, forgive me, and love me. I know that living a life of sin is outside of Your will, but it is so hard because I'm scared of who I will be without my sin. Please help me to look to You and the Bible for guidance. Please help me to turn away from my sin and turn instead to You. Thank You for loving me Father. Amen.

PY Day!
Go take a few minutes to relax and paint your nails or better yet, have someone else paint your nails!
Remember to enjoy the day because this is the day the Lord has made.

Week Six

Meal Plan

	Breakfast	Snack 1	Lunch	Snack 2	Supper
Monday	Boiled Egg with Avocado Toast*	YC*	Chef Salad*	YC*	Taco Salad*
Tuesday	Chocolate Smoothie*	Strawberries	Taco Salad Leftovers	Peanut Butter Yogurt*	Sheppard's Pie*
Wednesday	YC*	YC*	Shepherd's Pie Leftovers	YC*	Roasted Vegetables and Pork Chops*
Thursday	Boiled Egg with Avocado Toast	Peanut Butter Yogurt	Roasted Vegetables and Pork Chops Leftovers	Strawberries	Chicken Avocado Burritos*
Friday	Chocolate Smoothie	YC*	Chicken Avocado Burritos Leftovers	YC*	Feta Salad*
Saturday	YC*	Strawberries	Feta Salad Leftovers	Peanut Butter Yogurt	YC*
Sunday	YOUR Family Tradition	YC*	YC*	YC*	Eat Out

You are probably wondering what is with the short grocery list and all the Your Choice (YC*) days on the above meal plan. The last thing I want you to do after reading this book is say to yourself, "Now what?" Yes, I have written out every breakfast, snack, lunch, and supper idea for the past five weeks, but now that we are in the last week of this book it's time you started getting into a routine of creating your own meal plans for the week so you can continue your health journey after you read this book. Having you choose what you're going to eat on certain days is going to start weening you off relying just on this book for food ideas. You'll also see that the Willingham Tradition on Sundays is no more. Because now it will be your family's Sunday Breakfast Tradition! Remember this book wasn't a diet fad but a lifestyle change. Embrace the change and make it your own!

Grocery List

SPICES
RED PEPPER FLAKES
RANCH DRESSING
TACO SEASONING
CACAO POWDER
HONEY
CINNAMON
VANILLA EXTRACT
ACV
BEEF STOCK
WORCESTERSHIRE SAUCE
SALT
PEPPER
GROUND MUSTARD
PAPRIKA
FRESH ROSEMARY
COCONUT OIL
RASPBERRY VINAIGRETTE

PRODUCE
AVOCADO
SPINACH
ICEBERG LETTUCE
MIXED GREENS
CARROTS
BELL PEPPERS
SALSA
BANANAS
ZUCCHINI
STRAWBERRIES
11 OZ. FROZEN MIXED-VEGETABLES
ONION
GARLIC
LEMONS
POTATOES
TOMATO PASTE
VEGETABLES OF CHOICE
(SEE WEDNESDAY'S SUPPER)

PROTEIN
EGGS
DELI HAM
DELI TURKEY
BACON
2 LB. GROUND BEEF
NUT BUTTER
PORK CHOPS
2 PACKS CHICKEN BREAST

DAIRY
CHEDDAR CHEESE
MILK
SOUR CREAM
PLAIN GREEK YOGURT
BUTTER
FETA CHEESE CRUMBLES
SHREDDED MOZZARELLA CHEESE

Monday, Devotion 36- I'm Watching You

"Train up a child in the way he should go: and when he is old, he will not depart from it." Proverbs 22:6 KJV

"Direct your children onto the right path, and when they are older, they will not leave it." Proverbs 22:6 NLT Study Bible

My family enjoys doing anything outside. A few months ago, we were at the lake letting the kids play and fish on the bank when Adam cast his lure right into a tree. I was watching the scene take place a safe distance behind Adam so he wouldn't hear me laughing. What was even more hilarious than watching Adam waving his rod in the air trying to get the lure unstuck was that Reed, who had been right beside his daddy fishing this whole time, began to copy his daddy's every move. If Adam's rod went up, so did Reed's. It was so cute because Adam had no idea that his little side kick was watching and doing everything he was doing.

That got me thinking, you really never know who is watching you to see how you handle a situation, or how you dress, or how you talk, or act. Setting a Christian example for those you come in contact with on a daily basis is a vital part of living for Christ. You never know who you are going to impact in this walk of life. I mentioned in a previous devotion to find a Christian mentor to look up to and to try and model yourself after… What if someone has chosen YOU to be their mentor?

Are you setting a good example for others? What about for your children?

Father, People are watching me on a daily basis whether I'm aware of it or not. Please help me to set the right example for others and please help my walk with You become stronger with each passing day. In Your name I pray, Amen.

HD #5 on page 85 is your workout of today. Be the one that sets the example today and go workout!

Tuesday, Devotion 37- Mighty Hands

"That if thou shalt confess with thy mouth the Lord Jesus, and shalt believe in thine heart that God hath raised Him from the dead, thou shalt be saved." Romans 10:9 KJV

"If you confess with your mouth that Jesus is Lord and believe in your heart that God raised Him from the dead, you will be saved." Romans 10:9 NLT Study Bible

When you're feeling overwhelmed, depressed, upset, tired, anxious, or angry, the devil will try to keep you down by making you question your faith with questions like, am I really saved? Or does Jesus love me? The Scripture states many times that if you are truly saved then nothing or no one can pluck you from God's mighty hand (John 10:29). Chances are if you are a Christian and you are scared, worried, or depressed, it's because you haven't been giving your problems to God and you've not been praying about things like you should have. Isn't it an amazing feeling to know that even when we stumble or fall we are still in God's mighty hands?!

If you are not a Christian and you don't know Christ as your Lord and Savior, I urge you to look at the Roman Road of Salvation on page 109. Don't wait another day to be in God's hands.

Dear Lord, I can't express my gratitude enough for never letting me fall from Your hands. I know I feel so much better about everything when I come to You in prayer and when I read my Bible. Please help me to stay on track with a daily fellowship time with You and help all those around the world that don't know You as their personal savior. Amen.

LD #4 Is today's workout on page 90.

Wednesday, Devotion 38- Make it Count

"But sanctify the Lord God in your hearts: and be ready always to give an answer to every man that asketh you a reason of the hope that is in you with meekness and fear:" 1 Peter 3:15 KJV

"Instead, you must worship Christ as Lord of your life. And if someone asks about your Christian hope, always be ready to explain it." 1 Peter 3:15 NLT Study Bible

There are 24 hours in a day. Once that 24 hours of that day has passed, you will never be able to get it back. The older I get the faster it seems Christmas comes and goes. It literally feels like yesterday when Adam was driving (over the speed limit) to get me to the hospital to have our first baby boy. You always hear "old" people say things like "time flies" or "it feels like yesterday" … well I guess that makes me (gasp!) an old person because I catch myself saying things like that all the time!

With time going by so fast it should make the Christian be that much more focused and committed to spreading the good news of Jesus Christ to others. We should always be on the lookout for an opportunity to share the gospel with someone. And when we get asked about our faith or why we are acting differently the Bible tells us to be ready to explain our reason for hope. Don't let the next 24 hours go by without mentioning God to someone.

Father, Thank You for blessing me with the time I've already had here on earth. Please forgive me for not taking all the opportunities I've had to share the good news to others. Please allow doors to be opened so that I can share about Your love to someone and help give me the words to witness to them and explain why I have hope. Please go with me through the rest of the day and keep me safe as I ____________________________ in Jesus' name, Amen.

HD # 6 is your workout for today which is on page 86. Be motivated and excited because by this point you should feel yourself getting strong physically and hopefully spiritually! Take this time to burn some fat and feel good about yourself!

Thursday, Devotion 39- Love Christ First

"But seek ye first the kingdom of God, and his righteousness; and all these things shall be added unto you." Matthew 6:33 KJV

"Seek the Kingdom of God above all else, and live righteously, and he will give you everything you need." Matthew 6:33 NLT Study Bible

On one of our rock climbing adventures I saw some graffiti spray painted on the side of the rock that read "Love Yourself First." I kept thinking about that graffiti the rest of that day because I strongly disagree with that statement. When you put yourself first then pride creeps into your heart and life. You feel like YOU are more important than other things going on around you. That YOU are smarter, better looking, and stronger. That YOU should have the nice new car because YOU work hard. Or that YOU should have more money and nicer things because YOU deserve it. This "you" thinking will slowly start to overpower your whole life and turn that pride into bitterness. There will become a void in your life and you will search frantically to find something that will fill that hole in your soul sin has caused.

However, nothing of this world can ever fill the void Christ is supposed to fill in your life. Drugs, alcohol, food, nice things: all this will only help and make you happy for a season. Then YOU will lose interest and go searching for other forms of happiness or be so consumed in the sin that you have no idea how to set yourself free. This is what happens when you put yourself first. But when you put Christ first and you strip your pride and you truly set your eyes on Him, mountains can be moved and you will feel the power of the Holy Spirit in your life helping you through each and every day. It's a power unlike any other power. You live your fullest life when Christ is first. Not yourself.

God, I need You, I've been seeking happiness through _________________ instead of looking to You. I have selfishly been putting myself first. Please help me to no longer see myself as number one, but You at your rightful place as number one in my life. I love You. In Jesus' name, Amen.

Okay here is another chance to let yourself grow and create a habit of planning your own workouts. Today is a YC* day which means you can pick a workout from this book, which starts on page 81, or you can get a workout from some other source. You can even go for a run instead of doing exercises if you'd like. Whatever you choose to do, get in a sweat!

Friday, Devotion 40- Finding Purpose

"And in very deed for this cause have I raised thee up, for to shew in thee my power; and that my name may be declared throughout all the earth." Exodus 9: 16 KJV

"But I have spared you for a purpose- to show you my power and to spread my fame throughout the earth." Exodus 9:16 NLT Study Bible

It is so easy to take the simple road in life and be a good person, but have no life purpose. God tells us that we all have a purpose and it doesn't just deal with us, but those that are around us as well. This could be co-workers, classmates, family members etc. Once you find your life's purpose, don't let anything stand in your way of fulfilling the purpose that God has laid before you. The devil will try many tactics such as procrastination, laziness, self-doubt, fear, and hate to obstruct you.

It's like the man standing at a crossroads, he can do one of three things. He can take the worldly, easier way that is more popular and although you're moving forward, you're not moving towards God.

The second thing this man could do is stay exactly where he's at. Never making progress in this life towards anything. This man's life is stalled and not what God intends us to do.

Or you can take the road less traveled. The road of your purpose, the road that follows God's will. That will be very hard, but will reap eternal benefits. My prayer is that if you are reading this today you've decided to take that road less traveled. You're picking up your cross and you are following God. Don't be okay with just being on the side of the road or even on the wrong road. Don't let anything come between you and your life's purpose.

Dear Lord, Help me to not only find my life's purpose but to pursue that purpose. I feel like I'm the man at the crossroads. Please take my hand and lead me down the right road. I want to follow You and please You. In Jesus' name, Amen.

HD #1 on page 81 is your workout for today. Go after it!!!

Saturday, Devotion 41- Tight Family

"But as for me and my house, we will serve the LORD." Joshua 24:15 KJV

"But as for me and my family, we will serve the LORD." Joshua 24:15 NLT Study Bible

If my family had a motto, this verse would be it. In today's world, the family is being ripped apart. Married couples that stay together are now a minority. Why? Because Christ is not the pillar of the relationship any longer. It's very easy with financial obligations, children, work, and hobbies to push God to the back burner. After all we can't even see Him, yet we can fully see that our child needs braces or that the house needs painted, or the television has the big game on.

Do you want me to let you in on a secret that's really not a secret? If you are living for Christ, you can see Him! Yep, that's right people you can actually see Christ!

I see Him every time my babies lay down at night and we are reading our Bible story as a family. I see Him when my toddler asks for specific prayer for a family member that I didn't even tell him to pray for. I see Him when there is a natural disaster and people and coming in from miles away, even different states, to help those they don't know. I see Him when I walk outside and feel the cool, crisp mornings when it's just me and nature. I see Him when a young man helps an elderly woman put her groceries in her car. I see Him when two men stand side by side despite the color of their skin and defend our country. I see Him when I am at church and the choir is singing and hands are raised up to the sky to give praise to our Lord… I see Christ. If you want to see Christ too it starts at home. Don't let the world rip your family apart. Pray together, spend time together, enjoy the little things. And most of all look for Christ in everything you do.

Come up with a motto for your family and write it down and place it somewhere you can see every day. It could be something you've lived by for a while or something you just came up with that you're going to start today!

Your grace and glory has no boundaries. Thank You, Father, for letting me feel Your presence in my heart and soul. Thank you for letting me see you in the world around me. Amen.

Whoo hoo who is excited about doing a FD today!? This is your last FD (of this book anyway), so I want you to rock it and have a blast. You can find the FD on page 91.

Sunday, Devotion 42- You Did It!

"Know ye not that they which run in a race run all, but one receiveth the prize? So run, that ye may obtain." 1 Corinthians 9:24 KJV

"Don't you realize that in a race everyone runs, but only one person gets the prize? So run to win!" 1 Corinthians 9:24 NLT Study Bible

I am so stinkin proud of you!!! You did it!!! (In my most southern voice as my hands are raised, with confetti and *Rocky* music playing in the background.)

I'm sure there have been many ups and downs during this six weeks but you ran the race and for that you should be so very proud! I want to encourage you to not just run the race, but run the race to win! Go for your goals. If you met them, then that's absolutely amazing! Make new goals and go after those! If you didn't reach all your goals this time around, it's okay, don't beat yourself up over it. Get back out there and train spiritually and physically until you do reach your goals.

A lot of people may be a little hesitant about what to do now that this six weeks is up. Well my sweet friends, I have made for you your very own meal planning page, workout page, and grocery list page that you can find in the back of this book. All you have to do is tear it out and make copies or just follow them as a guide and create your own. Just fill in the blanks and you'll be great! Remember that's why I had you start doing more YC* days, so that you could become your own advocate and continue to train your mind, body, and spirt for the race of life. I pray for you all daily. Remember that you're never alone.

I'd love to hear your story! Follow me on Instagram @getrealwithJess to continue to get motivation and encouragement from myself and others that want to build each other up spiritually. Looking forward to hearing from you!

In Christ,
Jessi

Read 1 Corinthians 9:24-27 to get inspired to continue getting fit for Jesus.

Remember to complete the Final Survey on page 78 and look at where you were six weeks ago compared to where you are now in your life!

Father, Give me the courage and strength to continue this journey of betterment. Help me to train my mind, body, and soul so that when the devil comes at me I'll be ready and so that I can honor You in all I do. Thank You for allowing me to complete this six weeks, but Father please don't let it end there. Use me how You see fit and help me to always strive to be better than I was yesterday. Amen.

Okay folks, to really treat yourself for finishing this journey, I want tonight's PY session to be a YC* PY. That means that you can pick out a PY night you've already done in the book or go make up something all your own. Just enjoy and pat yourself on the back for doing an awesome job this six weeks.

Final Survey

I am so proud of you! YOU DID IT! Six weeks have come and gone, do you remember the first survey you took before you started this health and fitness journey? Well now here's another one. Don't look at the old one until you have finished filling this one out then compare how you feel now to how you felt back then. Let's take a look about how you grew:

Age:

Height:

Weight:

What did you get out of this six-week program concerning your body (i.e. did you lose weight? Can you now walk up those stairs?)

What did you get out of this six-week program concerning your spiritual life? Have you become closer to God?

Circle the best answer that describes you at this time:

When I think of food…
G)   I think about how God made it as fuel for my body
H)   I feel like I have an eating disorder
I)   I get depressed because I know it will only turn to fat
J)   I must be stressed
K)   I think maybe it will make me happy if I eat something
L)   Other: _______________________________

When I think about working out…
g)   I think it's only for skinny people who are already in shape
h)   I don't think I have time
i)   I don't- I don't enjoy working out
j)   I feel like it gives me energy to accomplish Gods work
k)   I sort of feel like working out because I know it's good for me
l)   Other: _______________________________

My walk with God is…
g)   Struggling
h)   Non-existent
i)   Strained, I don't give him the time He deserves
j)   Great
k)   Better than it once was
l)   Other: _______________________________

Write out your 3 short-term goals again and explain if you reached those goals.
1. _______________________________
2. _______________________________
3. _______________________________

Have your long-term goals changed? If so write them down again.
1. _______________________________
2. _______________________________
3. _______________________________

Prioritize the following 1 being most important in your life right now and 15 being least important

___financial wealth
___family
___friends, my social status
___God
___working out
___eating a well-balanced diet
___my spouse
___my career
___my car
___my house
___my prayer life
___how others see me
___how I look
___how I feel
___my clothes

Picture time! Take a picture of the front of your body, side view, back view, then of the same fun pose you took before. Try to be in the same clothing and go back and compare the pictures from six weeks ago.

Here's the fitness test again! Let's see if you've gotten stronger. Put 30 seconds on a stop watch and see how many squats, pushups, and crunches you can do in the allotted amount of time.

30 second squats _______________
30 seconds of pushups _______________
30 seconds of crunches _______________

YAY YAY YAY! You're done! Go reward yourself with some healthy cookie dough and remember this book may be over but don't let that be the end of your story! Be your own advocate, remember the tips and tricks you've learned along the journey and most importantly remember to give it all to God!

Lord God, Thank You! Thank You for your grace, glory, love, and just being there with me every step of the way on this six-week journey. Please help me to continue with my healthy habits so I can be a better person for those that I love the most and to help further Your Kingdom. In Jesus' name, Amen.

Workouts

My workouts are designed so that you don't need any equipment unless you want to. By utilizing your body weight, you get a strong lean muscular physique along with increasing your energy level, fat burning metabolism, and endurance. Grab a mat and a timer to get started. Remember to stretch and warm up a little before completing any type of vigorous workout to prevent injury. Also make sure you are healthy enough to partake in such activity. If you feel like you need a break, take a break. Listen to your body and remember it's not about outdoing someone else's achievements, it's about outdoing your achievements; the only person you should be comparing to is yourself.

HD #1 perform each exercise for 30 seconds, rest when you need to, but try to complete an entire circuit before stopping. Ready to burn some fat? Let's go!!!

1.   Skaters

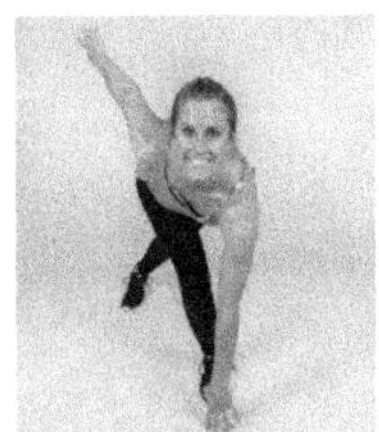 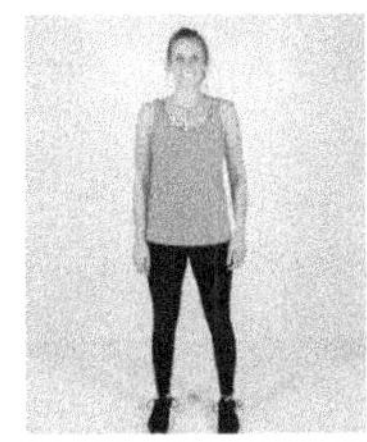 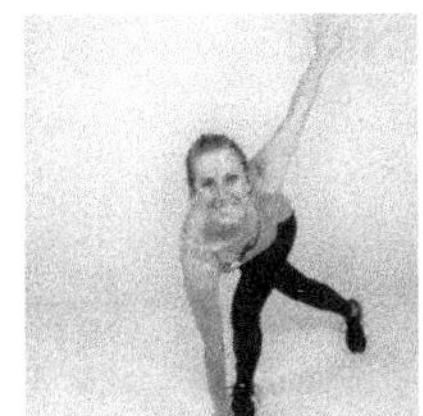

2.   Raised leg crunches

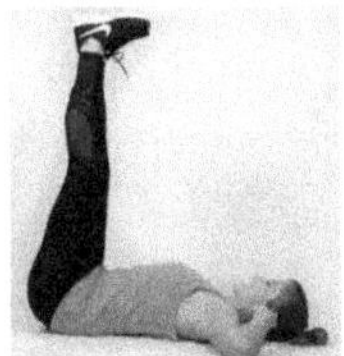 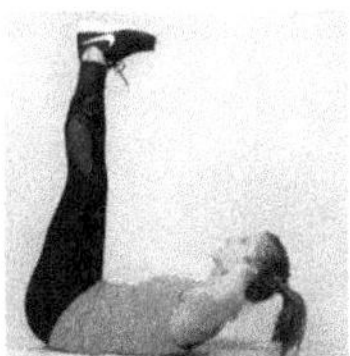

3.   Push up with an arm extension

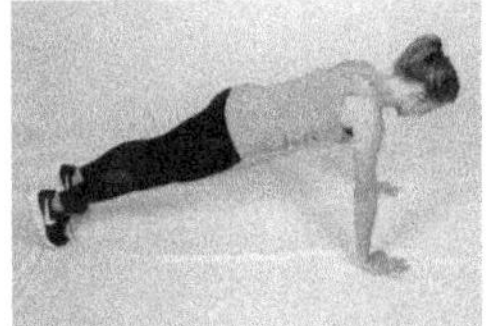 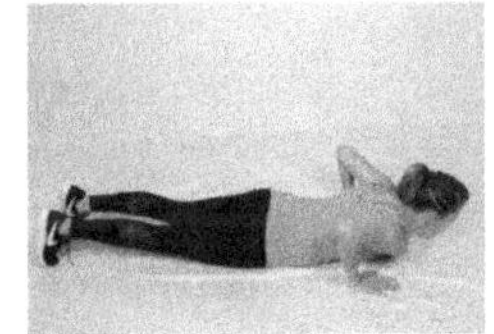 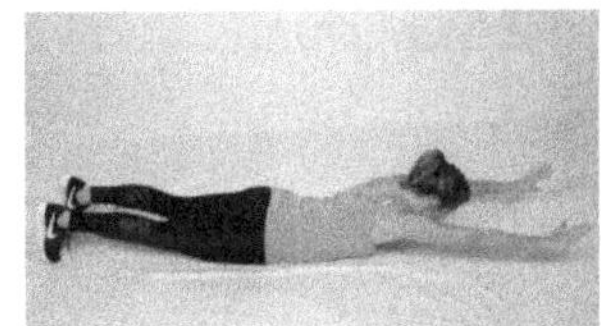

4.   Reverse lunge with a kick (alternate legs)

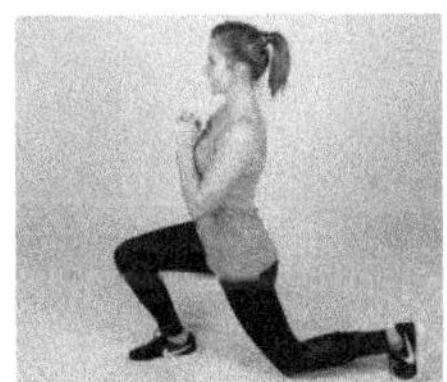 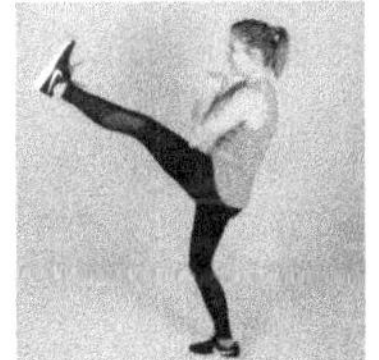

5.   Russian twists

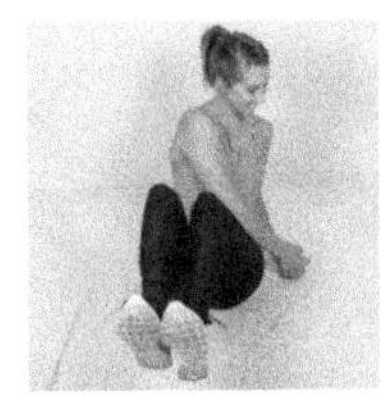 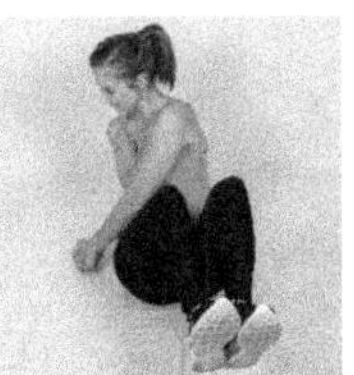

6.   Burpees

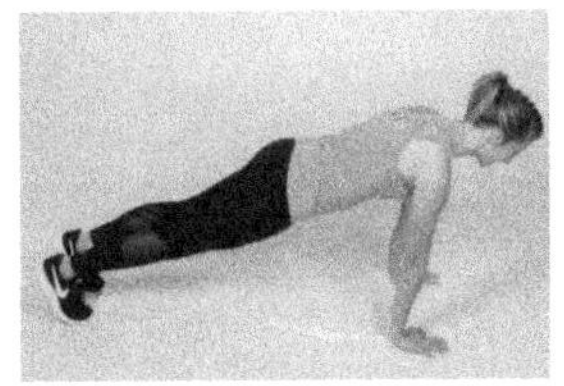 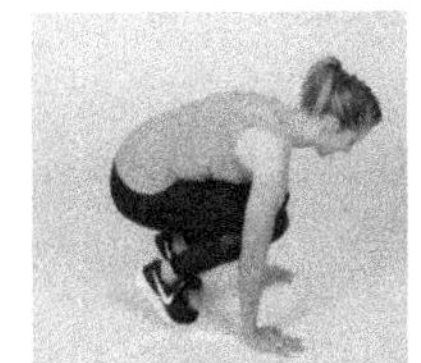 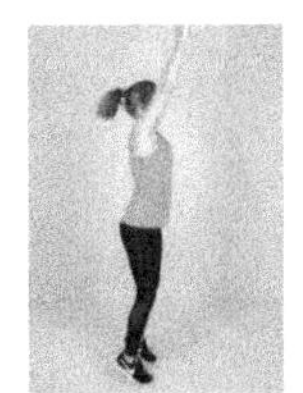 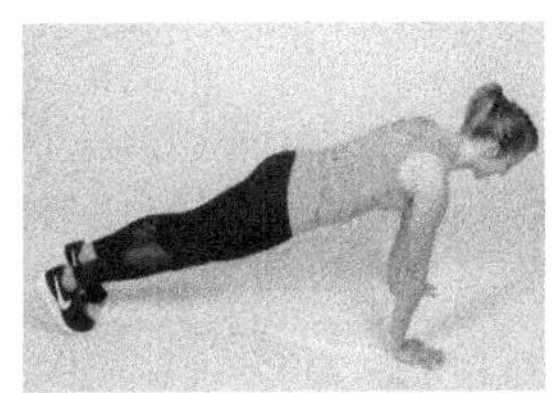

7.   1-minute rest. Repeat this circuit 3 more times for a total of 4 times.

HD #2 perform each exercise for 30 seconds, rest when you need to, but try to complete an entire circuit before stopping. Ready to burn some fat? Let's go!!!

1. Side Plank Raises- Left Side

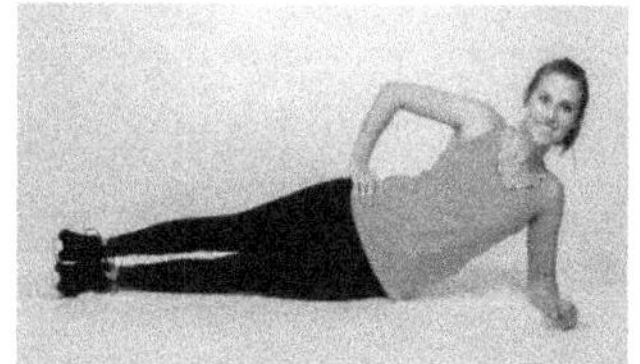 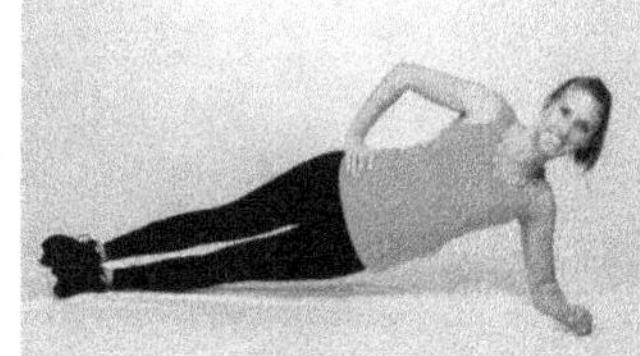

2. Side Plank Raises- Right Side

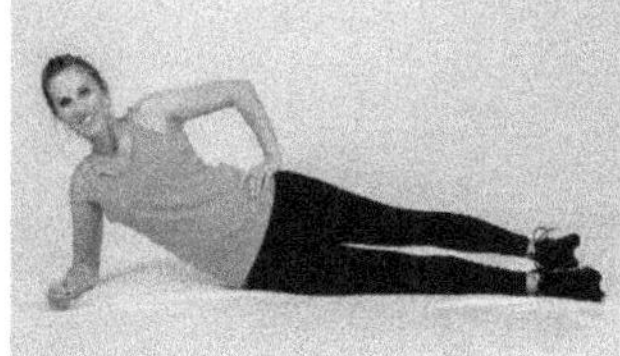 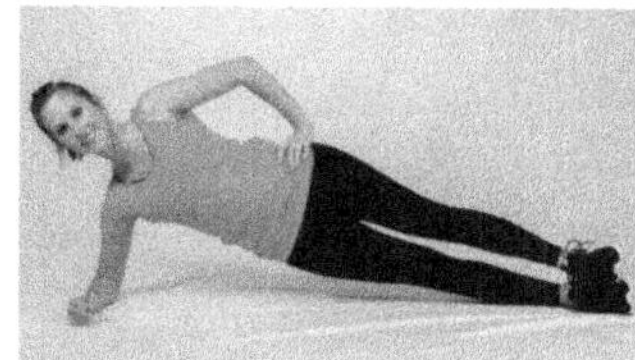

3. Three Count Supermans

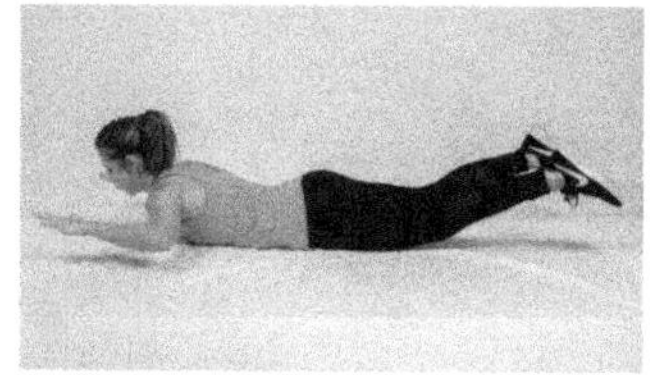 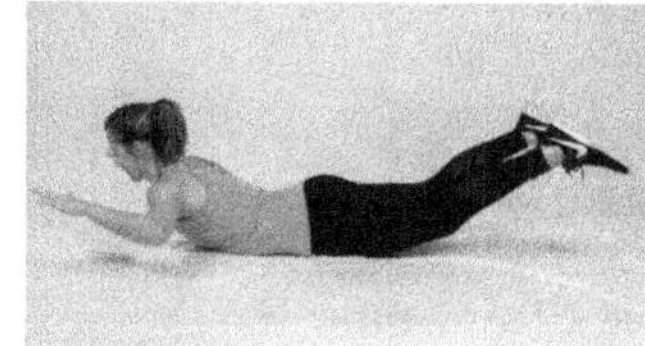 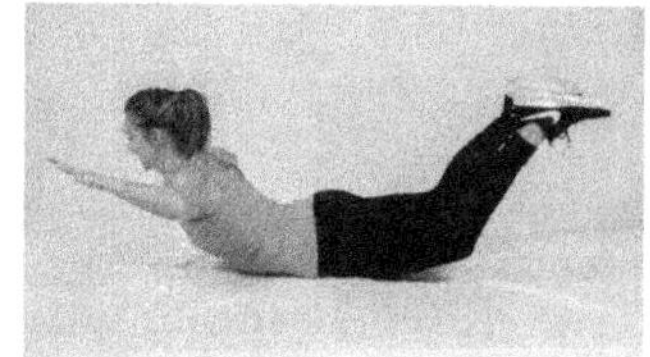

4. Bicycles

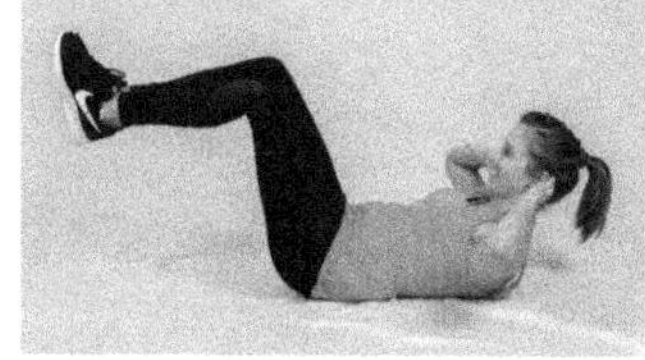 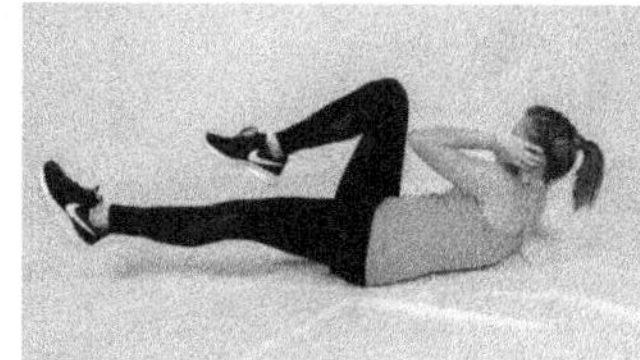 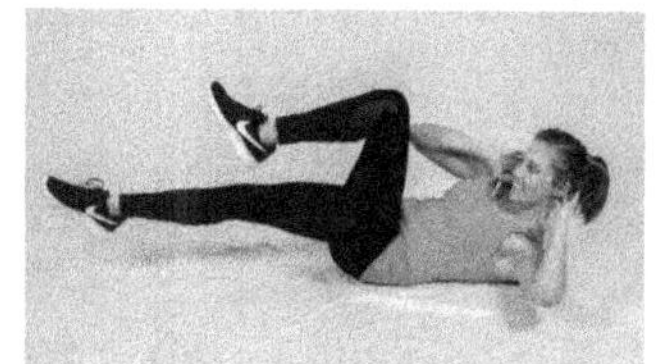

5. Frog Squats

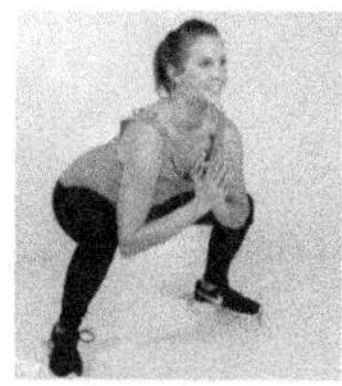 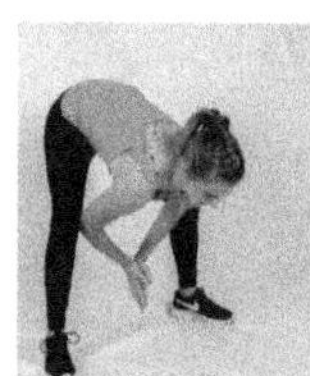 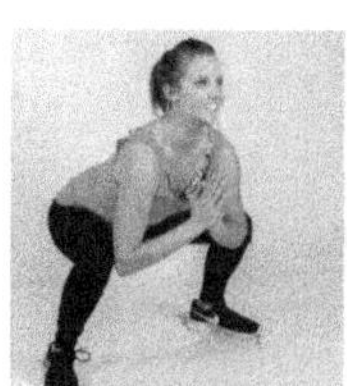

6. Scissor Kicks

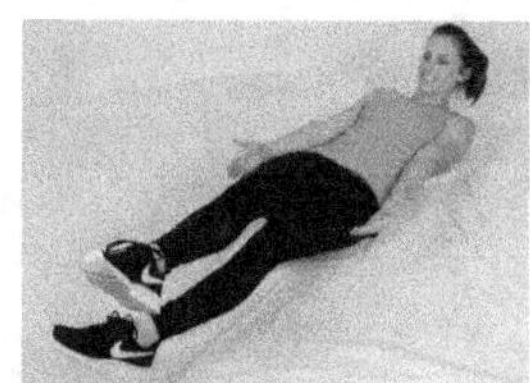 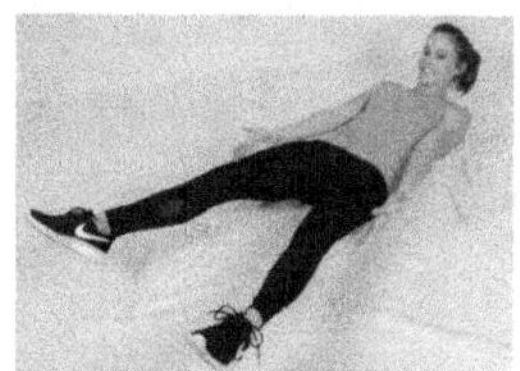 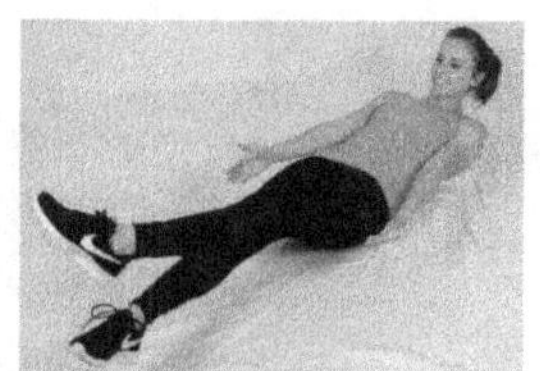

7. 1-minute rest. Repeat this circuit 3 more times for a total of 4 times.

HD #3 perform each exercise for 30 seconds, rest when you need to, but try to complete an entire circuit before stopping. Let's go!!!

1. Donkey Kicks (alternate legs)

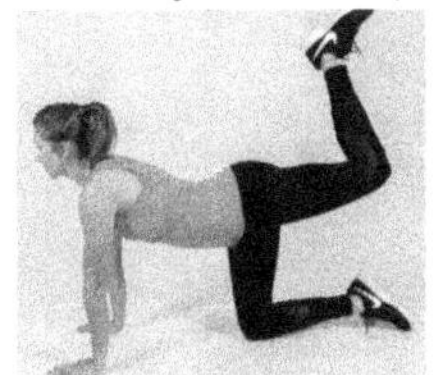 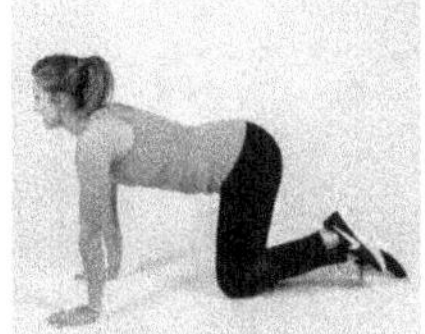

2. Jumping Jacks

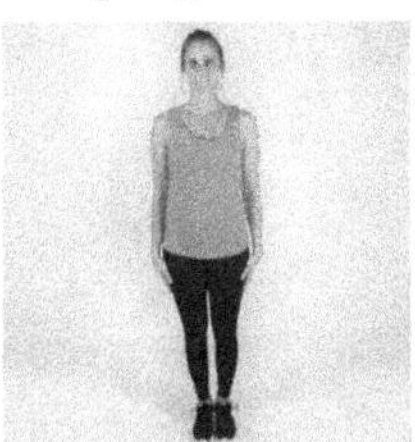 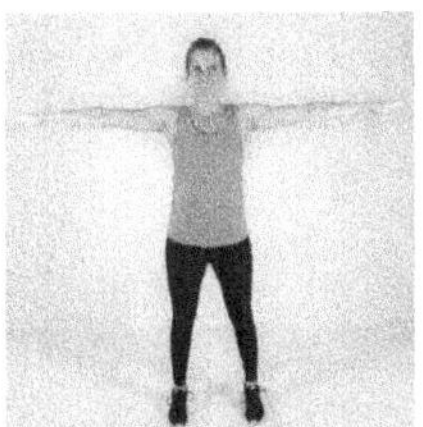 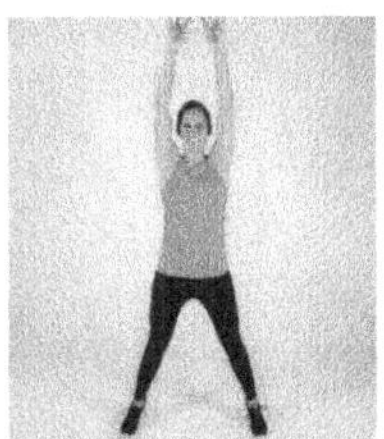

3. Mountain Climbers (Four Count) with Jack

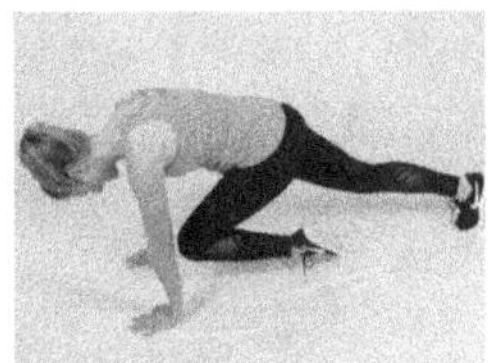 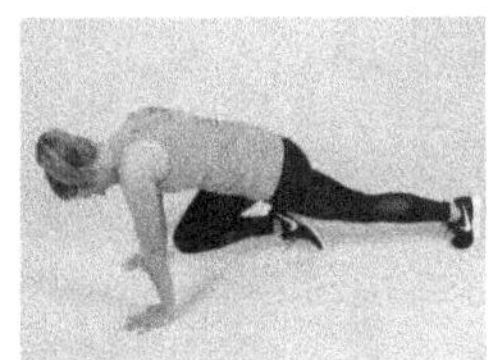 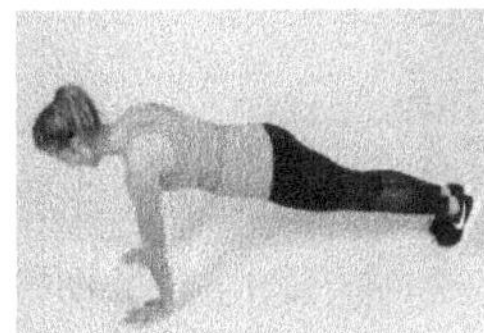 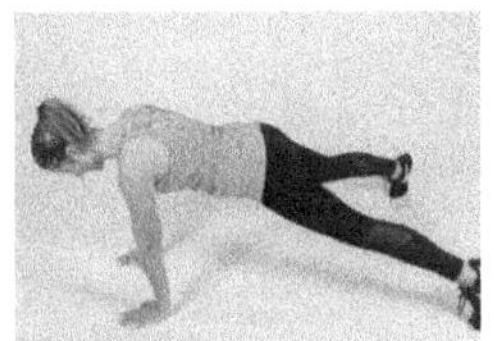

4. Floor Dips

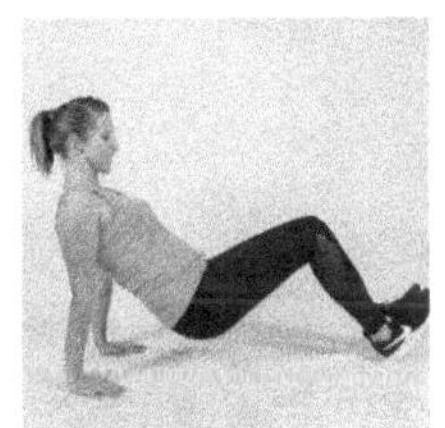 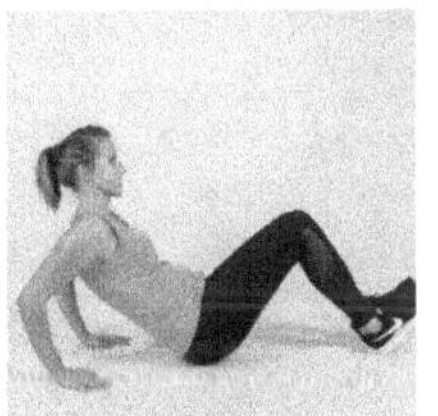

5. Jump Squats

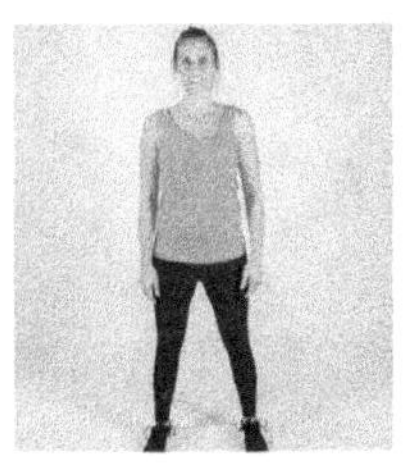 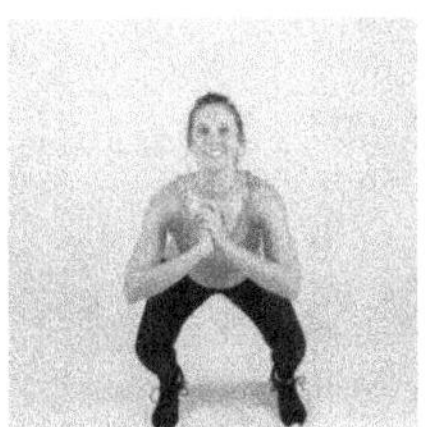 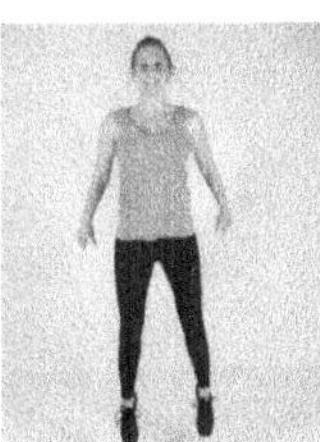

6. Dolphin Push Ups

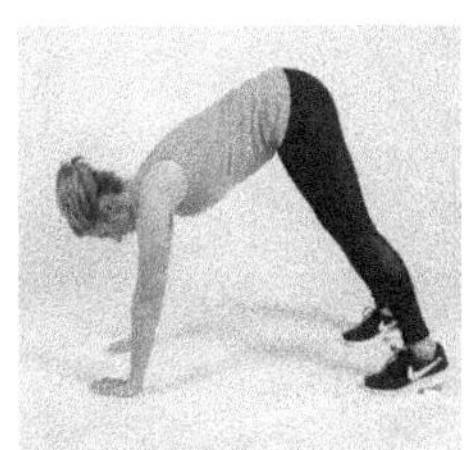 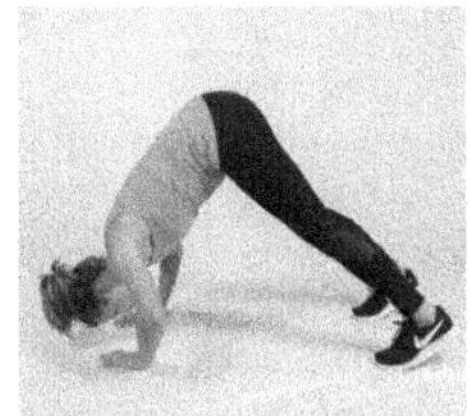

7. 1-minute rest. Repeat this circuit 3 more times for a total of 4 times.

HD #4 perform each exercise for 30 seconds, rest when you need to, but try to complete an entire circuit before stopping. Ready to burn some fat? Let's go!!!

1.   Plank with Alternating Hip Taps

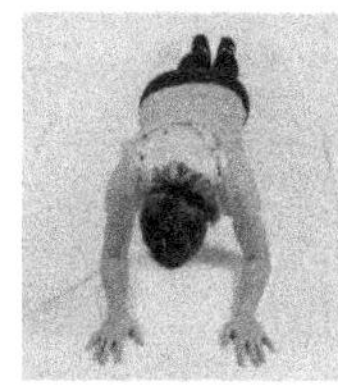 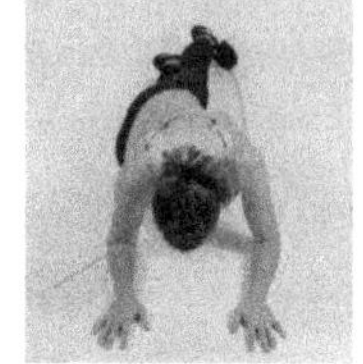 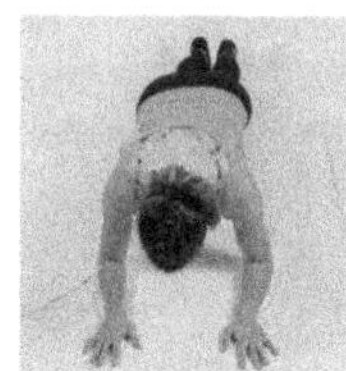 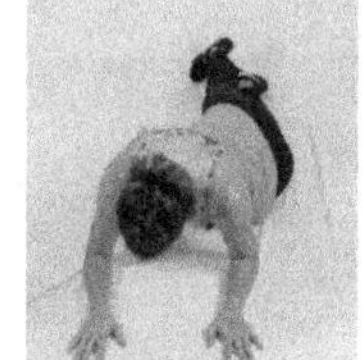

2.   High Knees

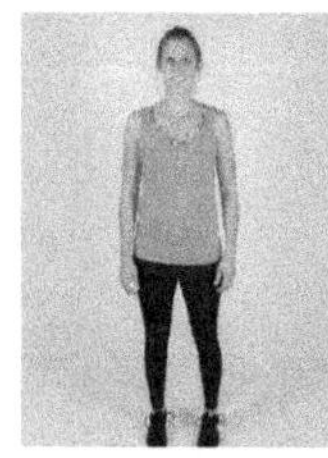 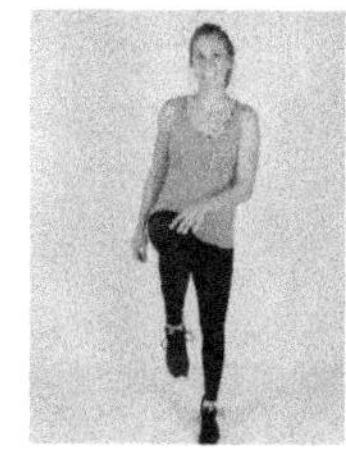 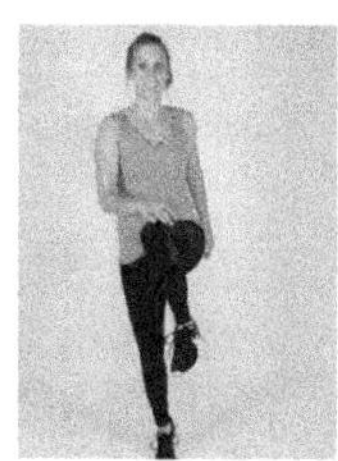

3.   Push up with Superman

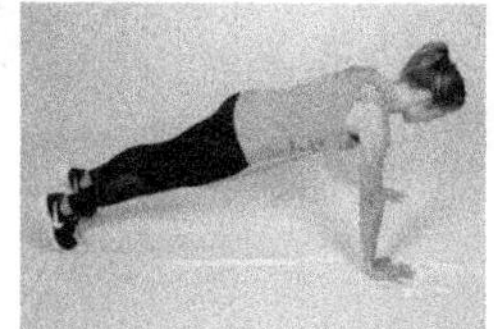 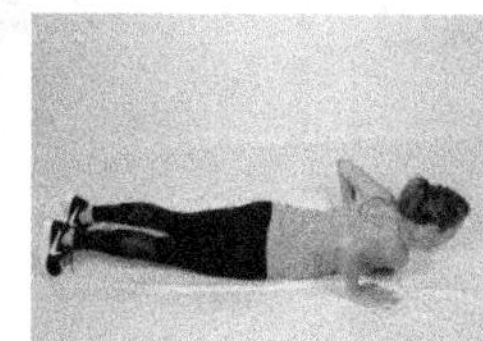 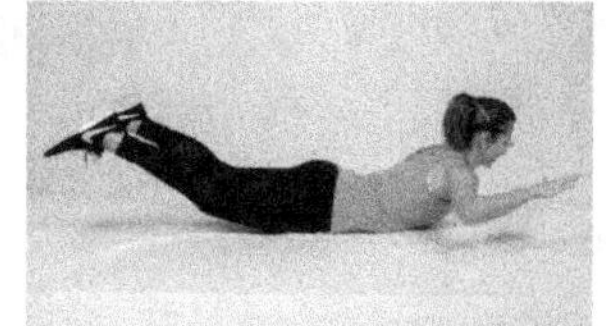

4.   Alternating Leg Raises

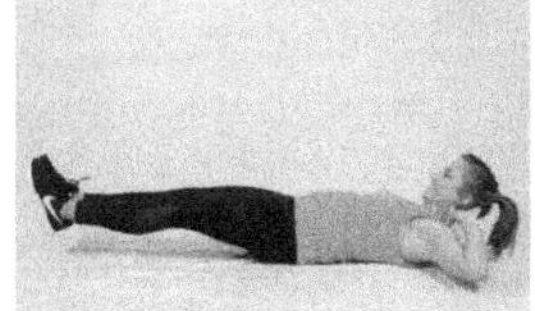 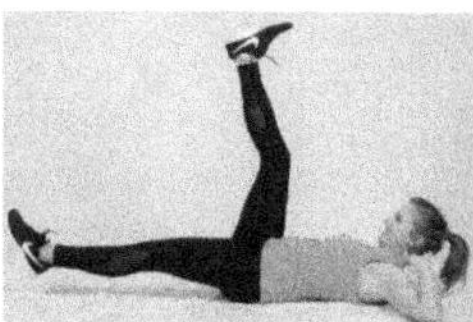 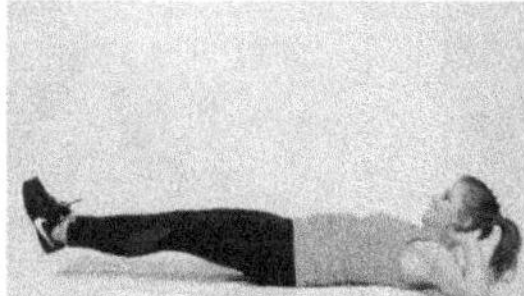 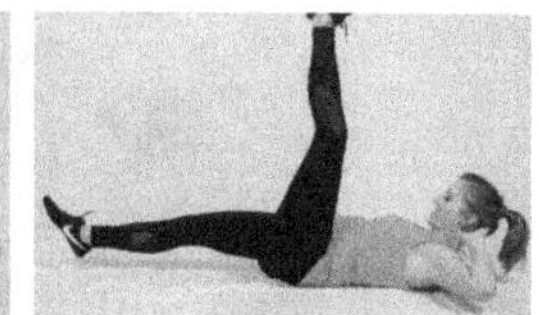

5.   Caterpillars

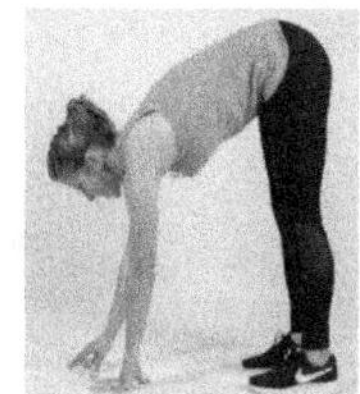 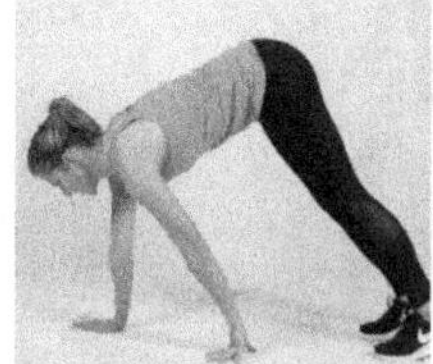 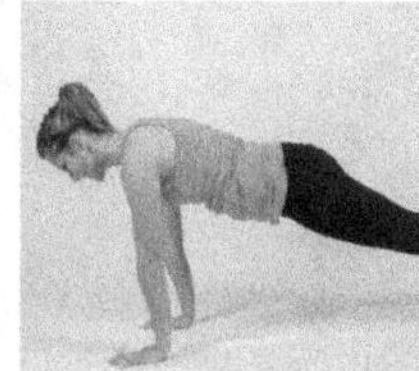 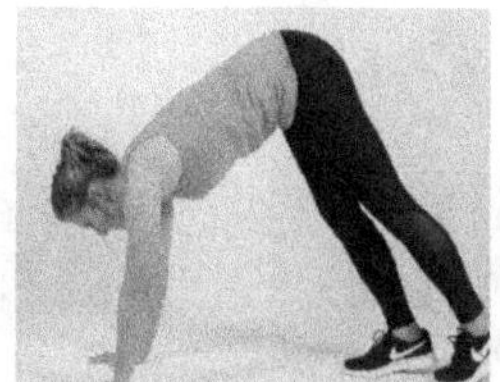 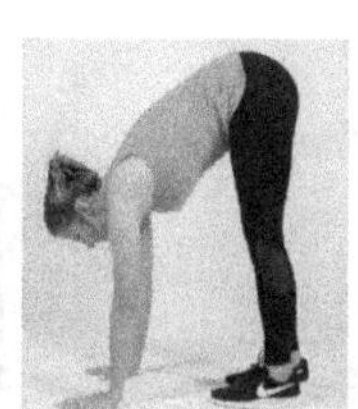

6.   Pulse Squats -In and Out- For Three Counts

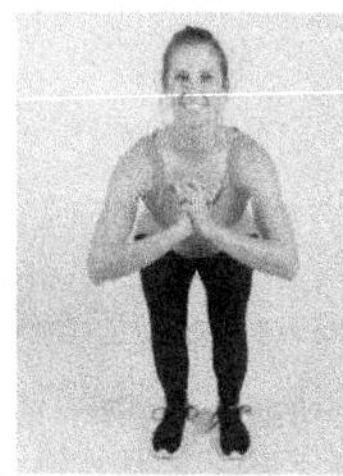 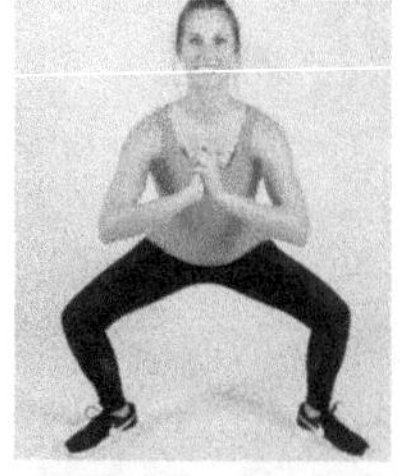

7.   1-minute rest. Repeat this circuit 3 more times for a total of 4 times.

HD #5 perform each exercise for 30 seconds, rest when you need to, but try to complete an entire circuit before stopping. Ready to burn some fat? Let's go!!!

1.   Alternating Lunges with Hip Extensions

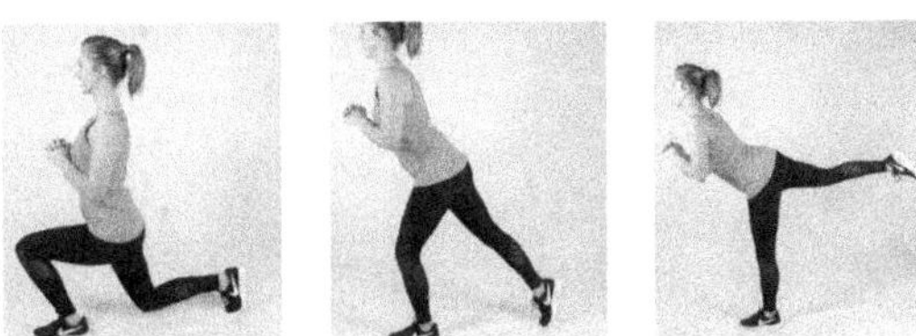

2.   Cross Body Crab Kicks

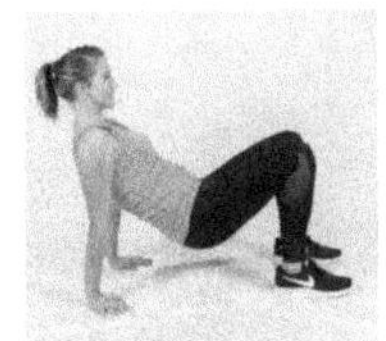 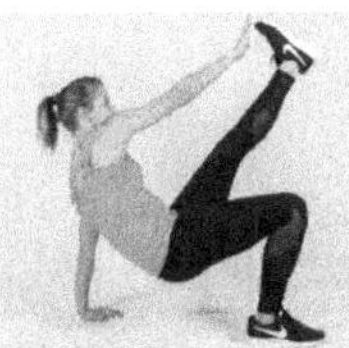 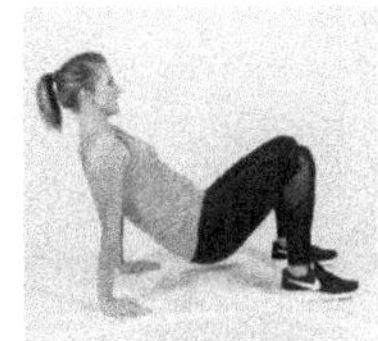 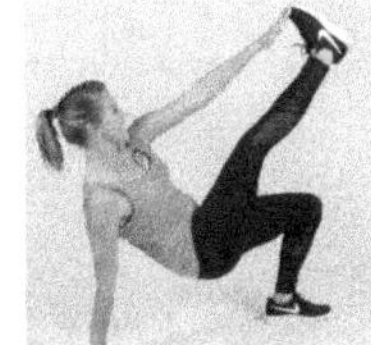

3.   Plank with Shoulder Taps

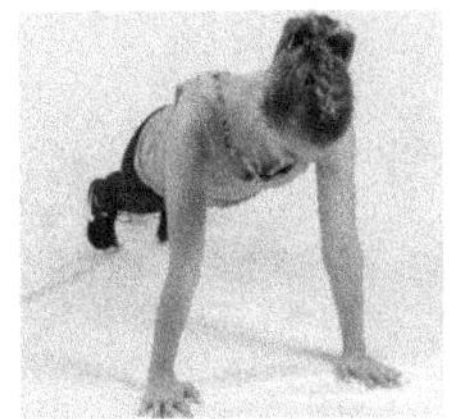 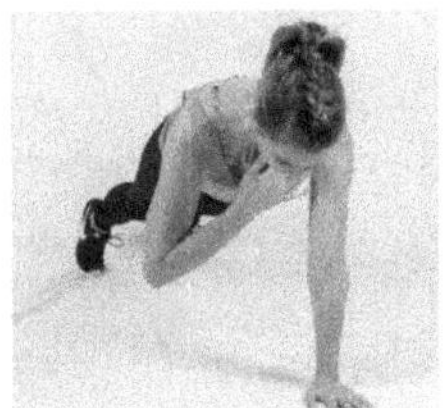 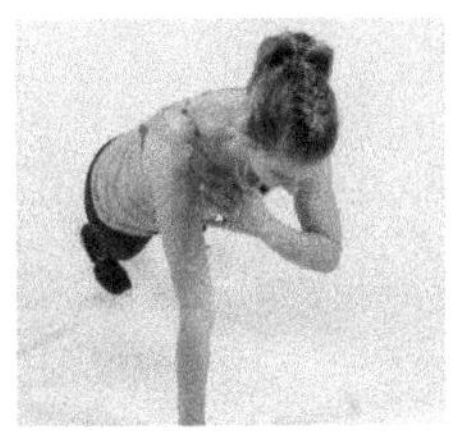

4.   Rainbows (alternate legs)

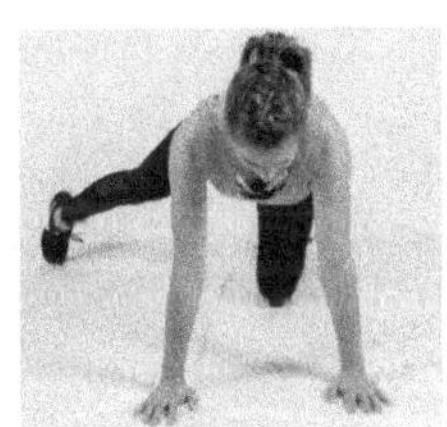 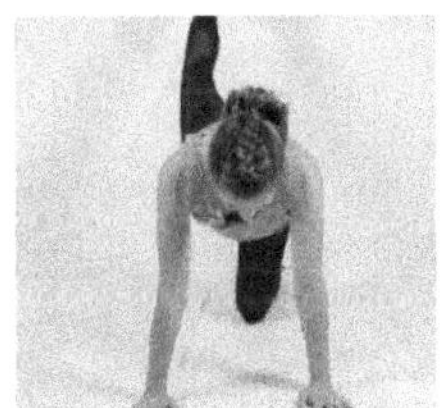 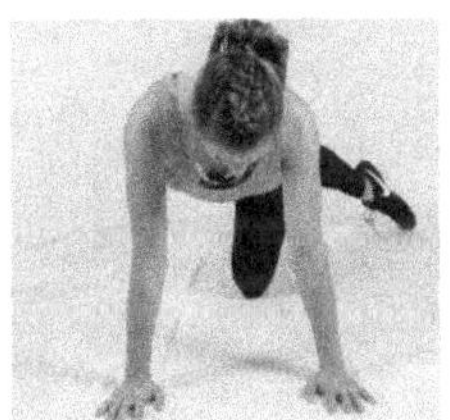

5.   Punches-As Fast As Possible

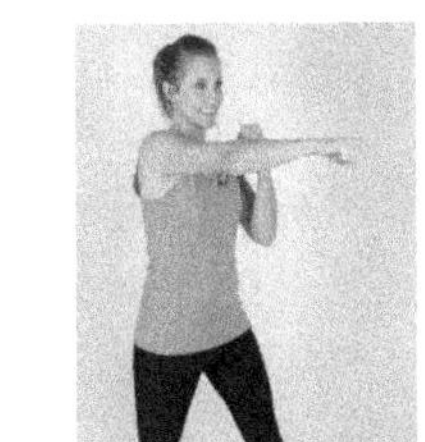 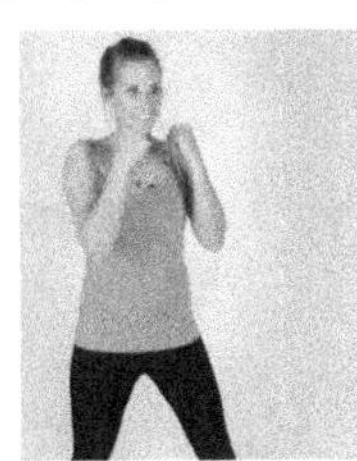 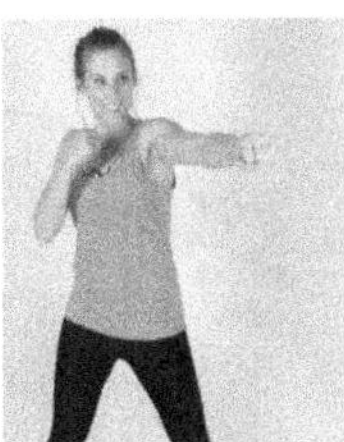

6.   Jumps with Knee Hits

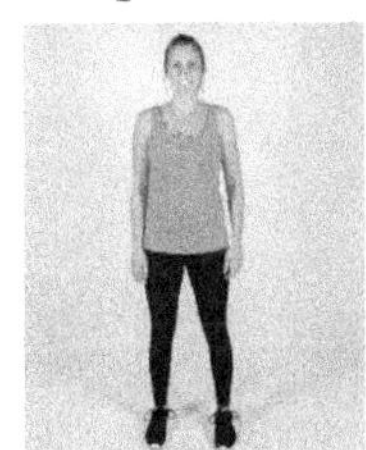 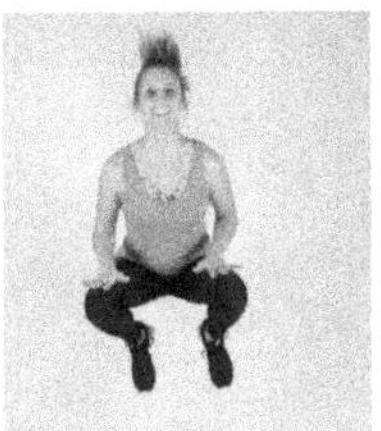

7.   1-minute rest. Repeat this circuit 3 more times for a total of 4 times.

HD #6 perform each exercise for 30 seconds, rest when you need to, but try to complete an entire circuit before stopping. Ready to burn some fat? Let's go!!!

1.   180 Jump with Burpee

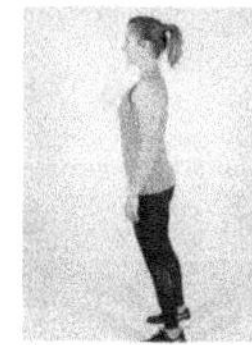 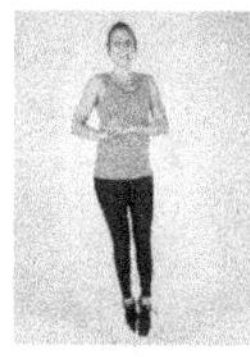 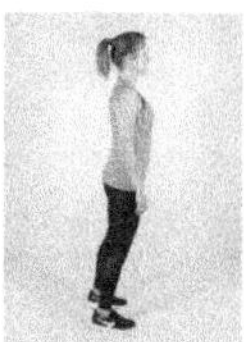 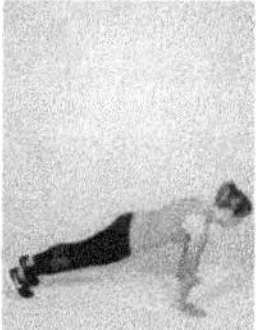 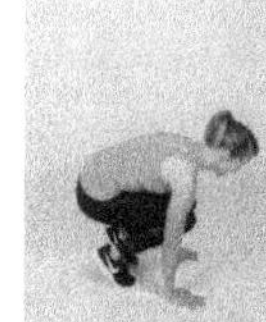 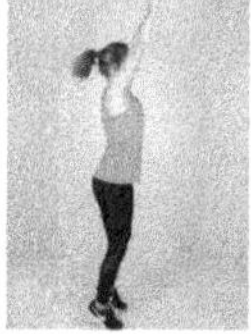

2.   Four High Knees Then Chest to the Floor

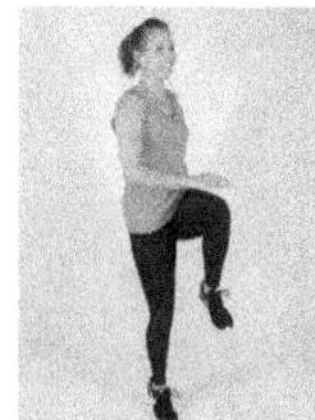 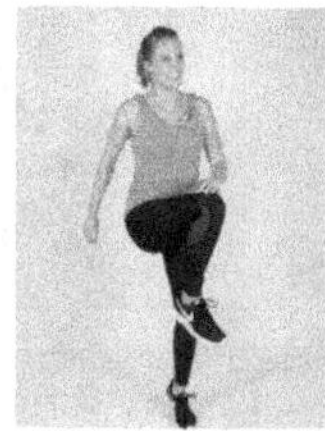 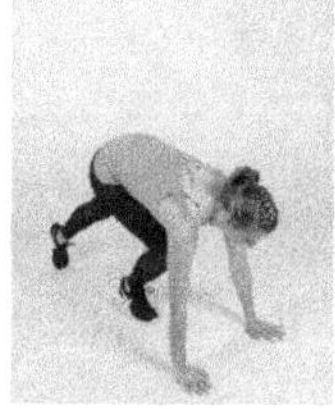 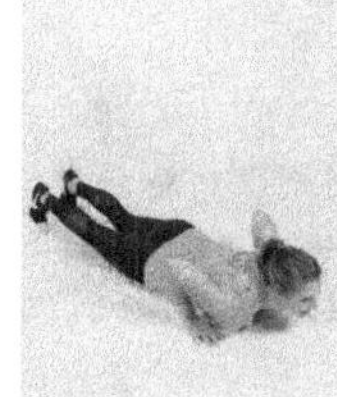

3.   Plank with Alternating Knee Taps

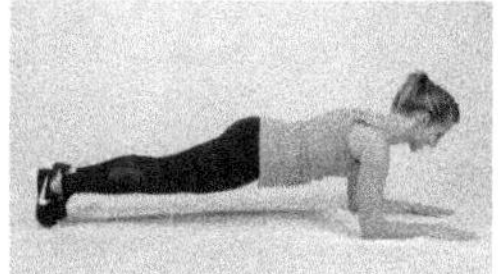 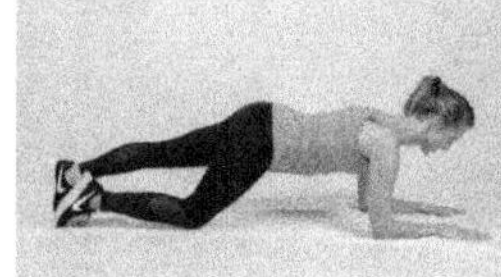 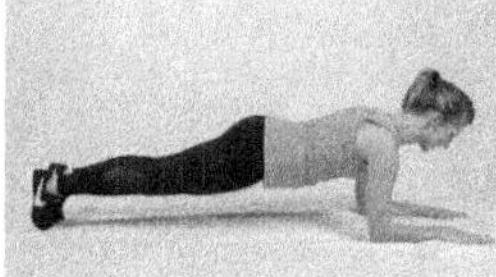 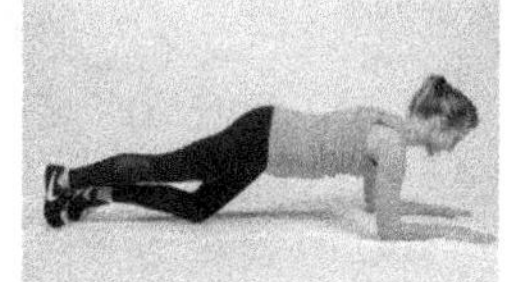

4.   Plank In and Outs

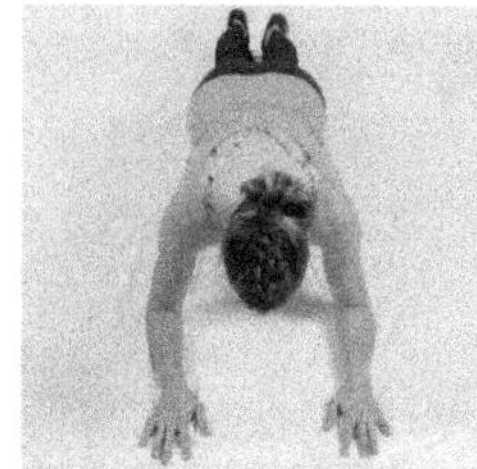 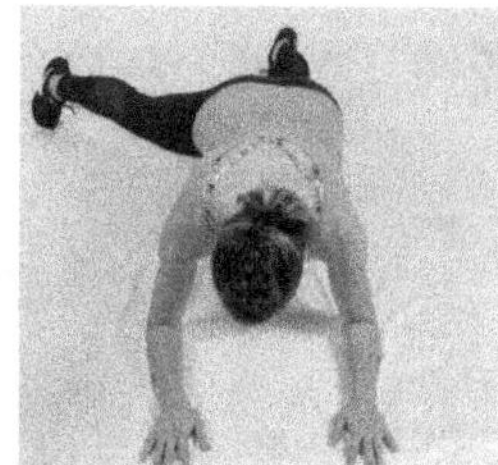 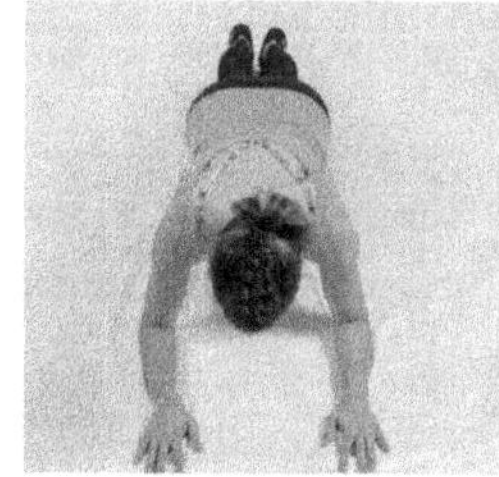 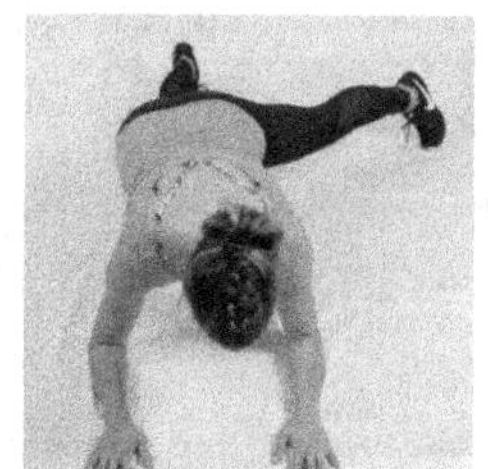

5.   Swimmers (continuously kick legs while arms are in circular motion)

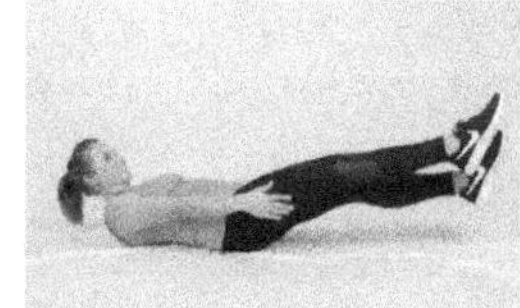 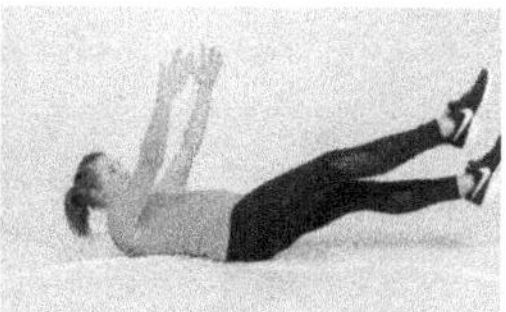 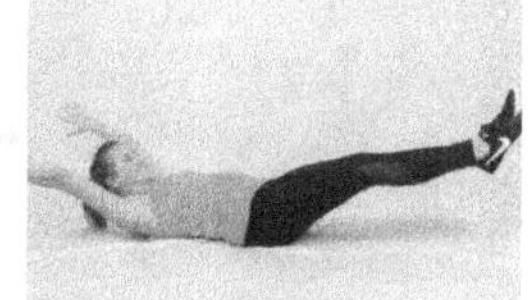 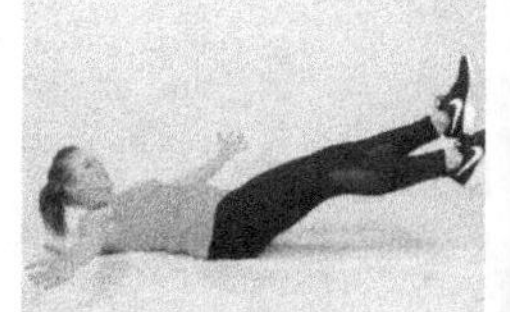

6.   Elbow to Hand Push Up (alternate pushing arm)

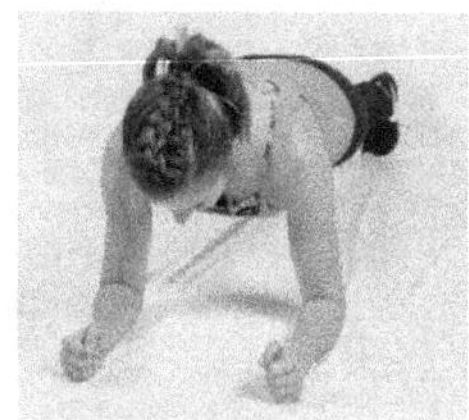 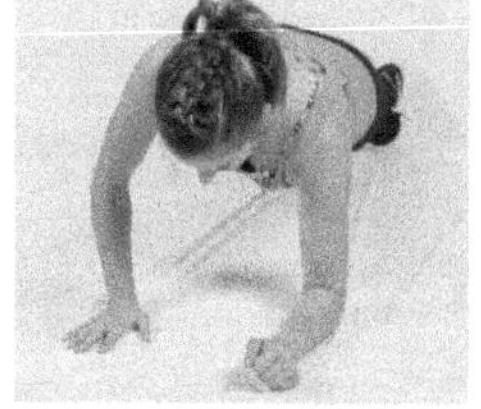 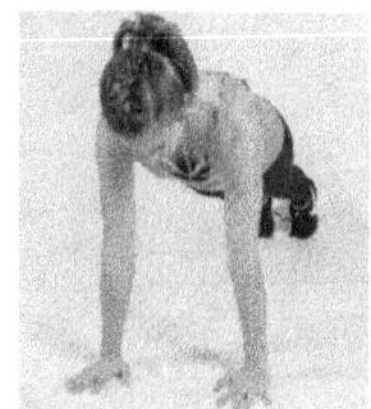

7.   1-minute rest. Repeat this circuit 3 more times for a total of 4 times.

LD #1 perform each exercise for 30 seconds, rest when you need to, but try to complete an entire circuit before stopping. Ready to burn some fat? Let's go!!!

1. Jog

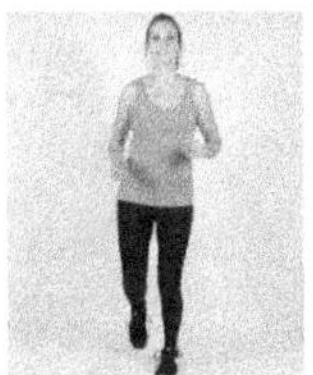 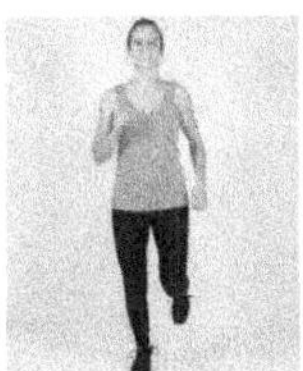

2. Jumping Jacks

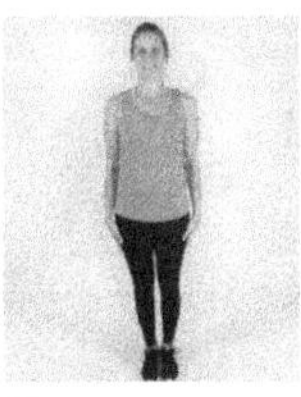 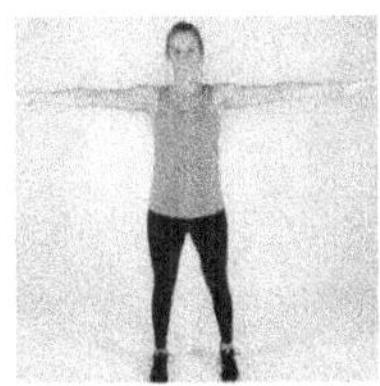 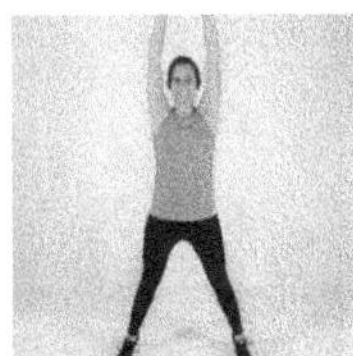

3. Jog

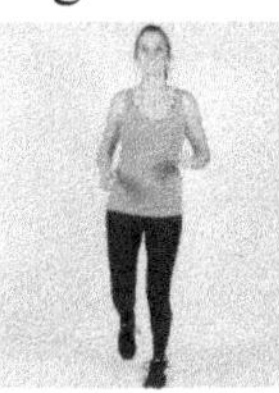 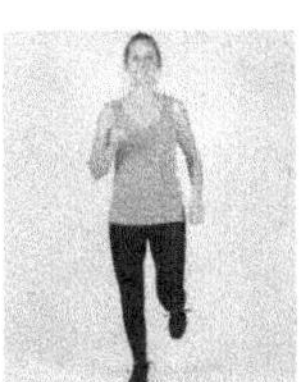

4. Jab, Jab, Uppercut, Uppercut

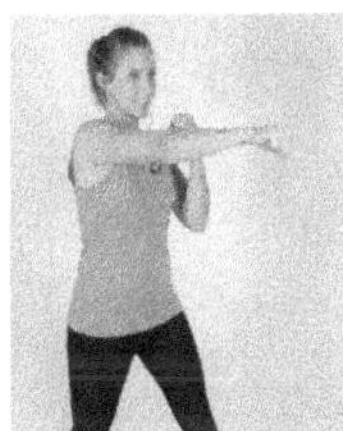 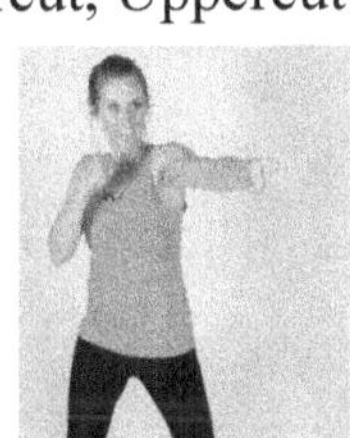 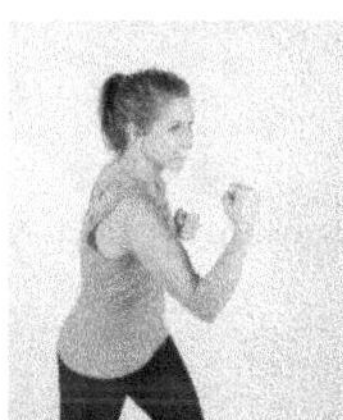 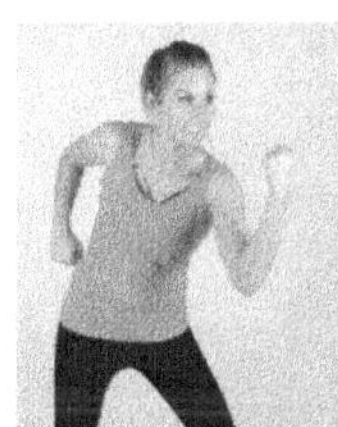

5. Jog

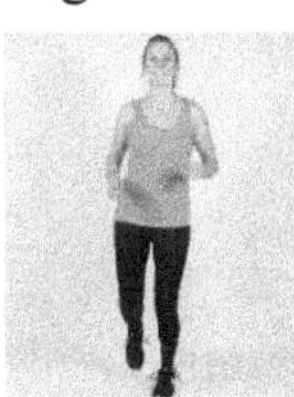 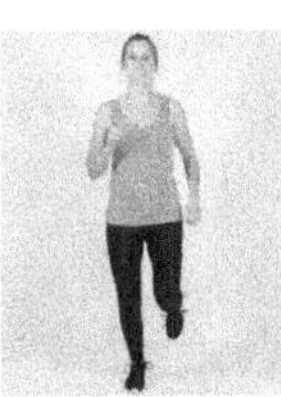

6. Side Knee to Elbow

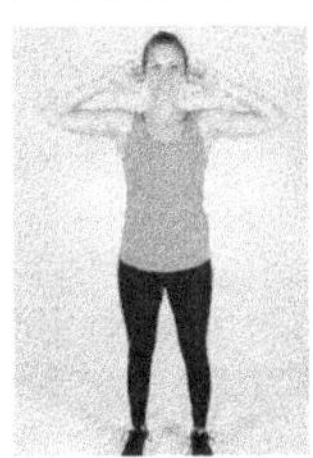 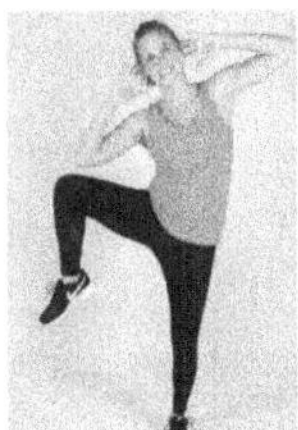 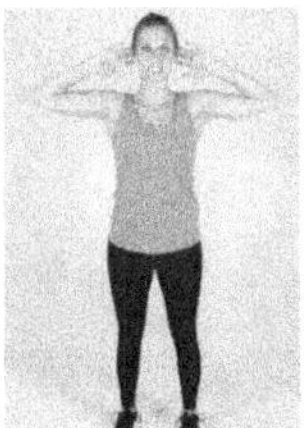 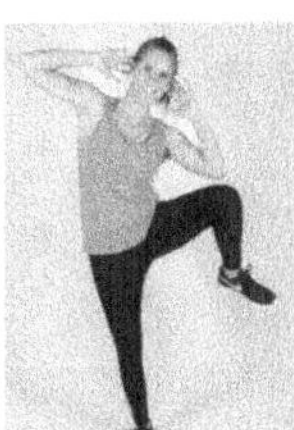

7. 1-minute rest. Repeat this circuit 2 more times for a total of 3 times. Once you have completed all three circuits put five minutes on your timer and stretch or perform yoga for that time. Really focus on elongating the body and relaxing the mind.

LD #2 perform each exercise for 30 seconds, rest when you need to, but try to complete an entire circuit before stopping. Ready to burn some fat? Let's go!!!

1.   Jog

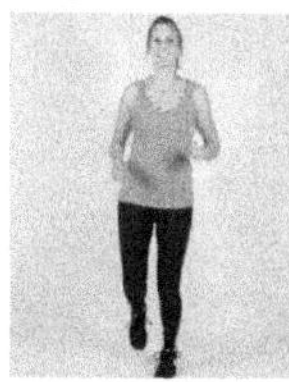 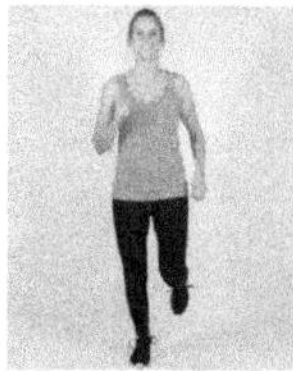

2.   Crunches

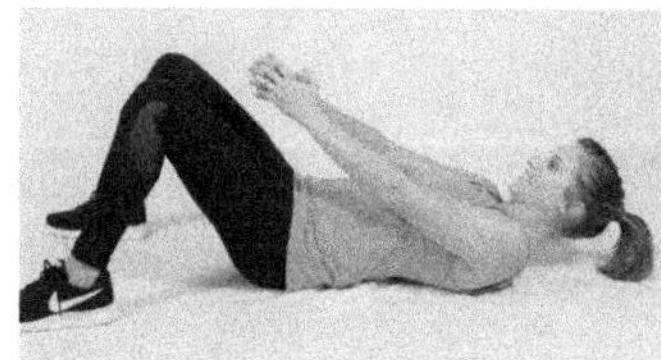 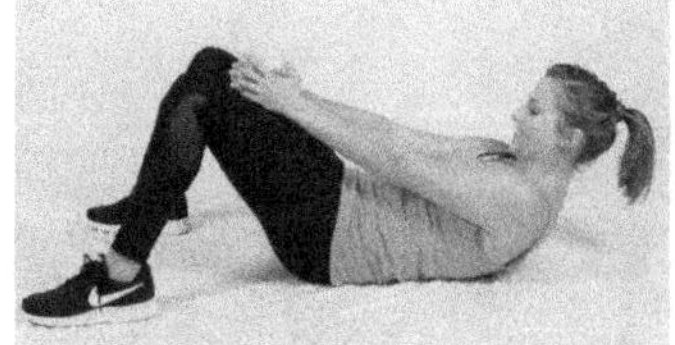

3.   Jog

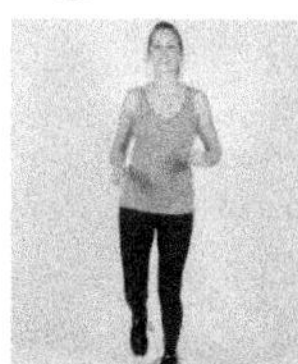 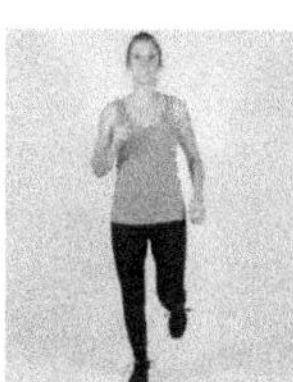

4.   Plank In and Outs

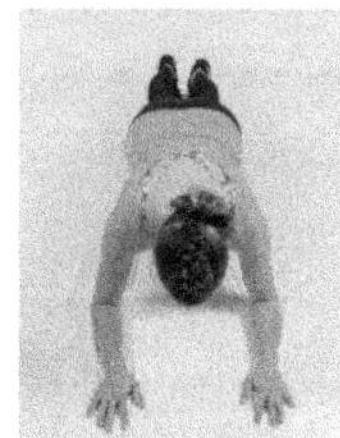 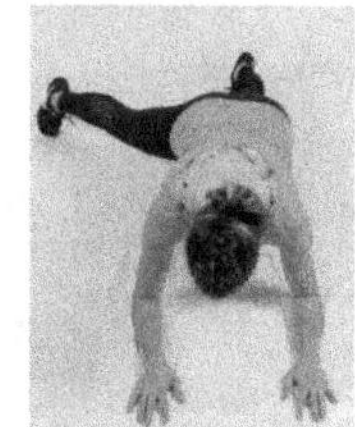 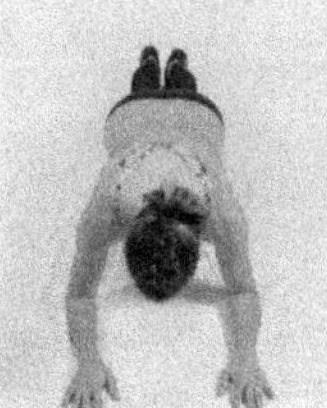 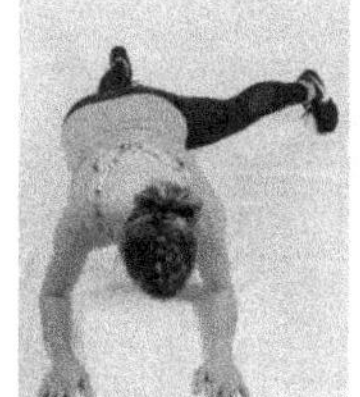

5.   Jog

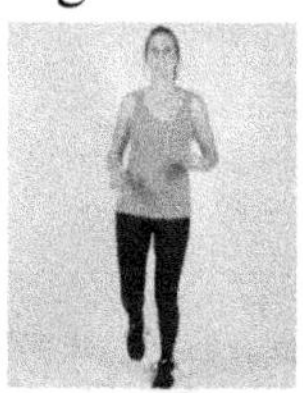 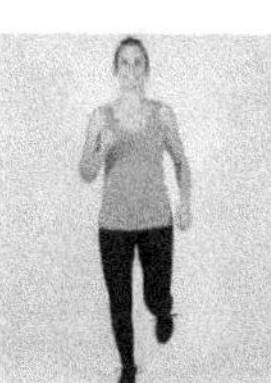

6.   Leg Climbers

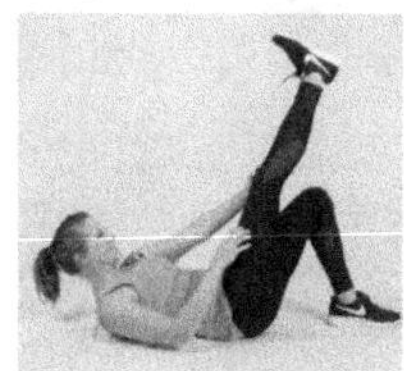 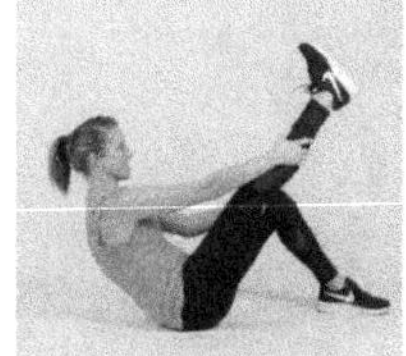 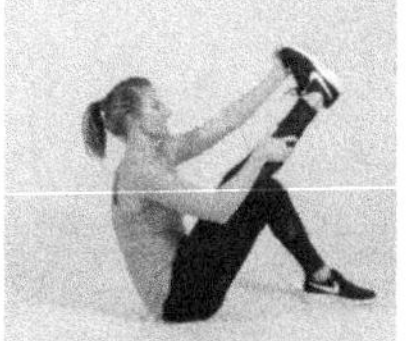

7.   1-minute rest. Repeat this circuit 2 more times for a total of 3 times. Once you have completed all three circuits put five minutes on your timer and stretch or perform yoga for that time. Really focus on elongating the body and relaxing the mind.

LD #3 perform each exercise for 30 seconds, rest when you need to, but try to complete an entire circuit before stopping. Ready to burn some fat? Let's go!!!

1.   Jog

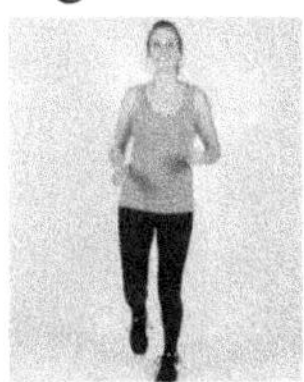 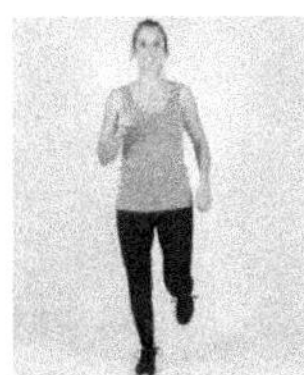

2.   Burpees

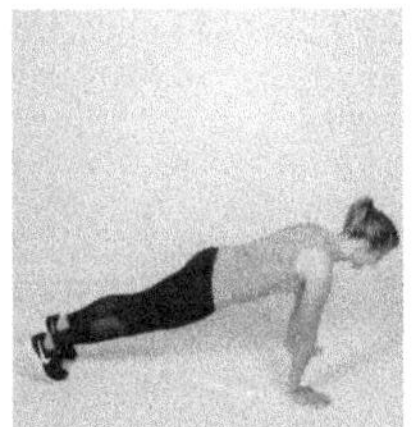 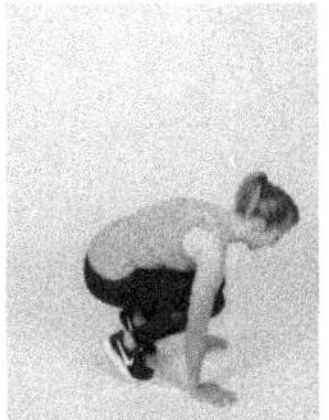 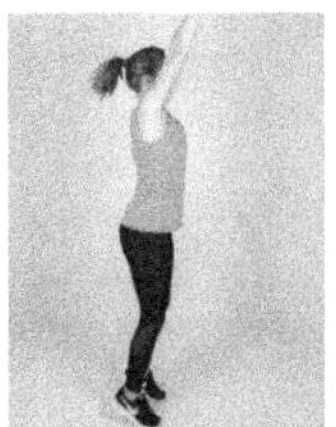 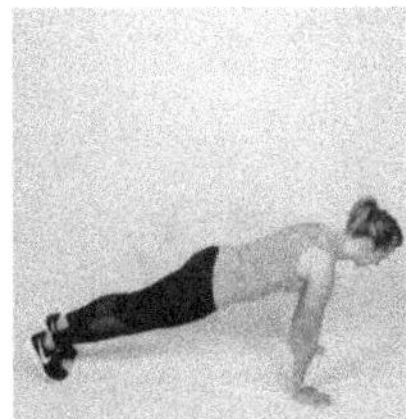

3.   Jog

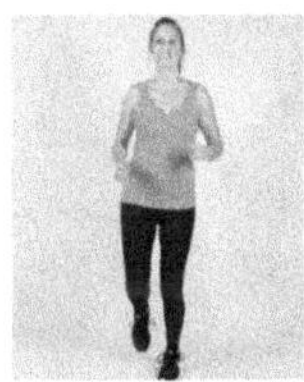 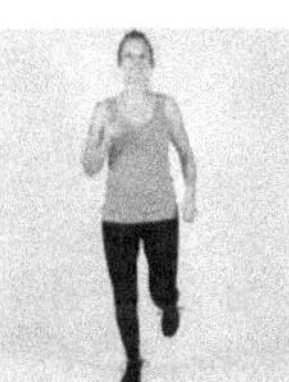

4.   Side Plank Raises- Left Side

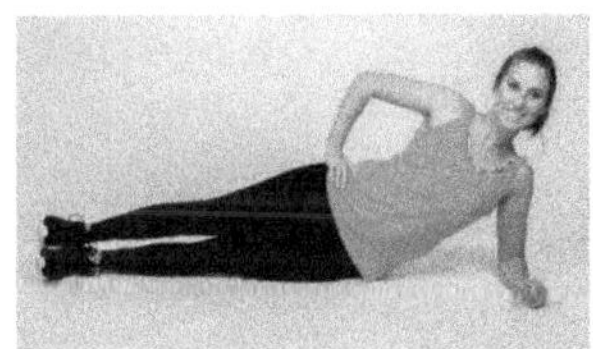 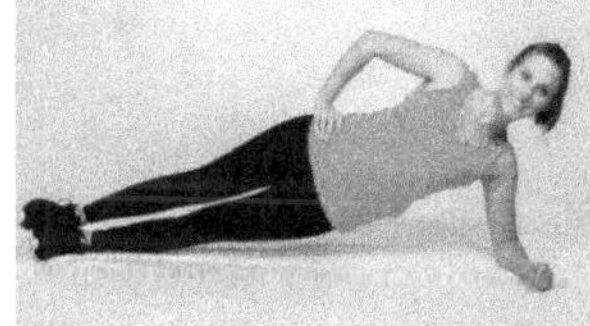

5.   Jog

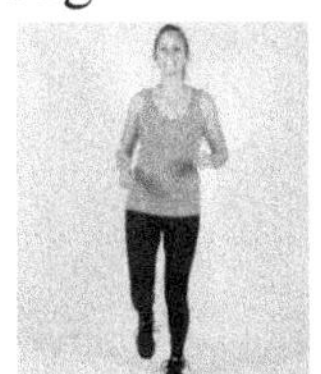 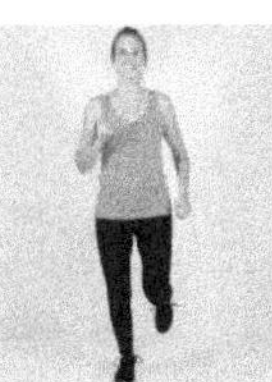

6.   Side Plank Raises- Right Side

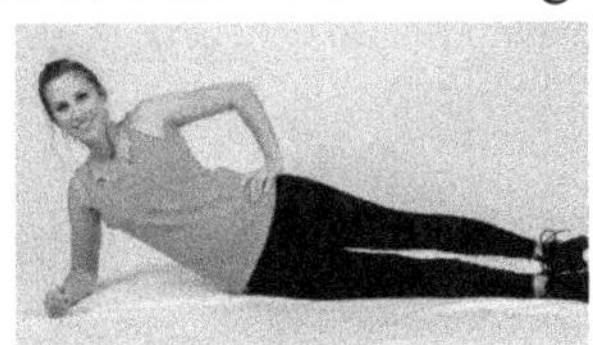 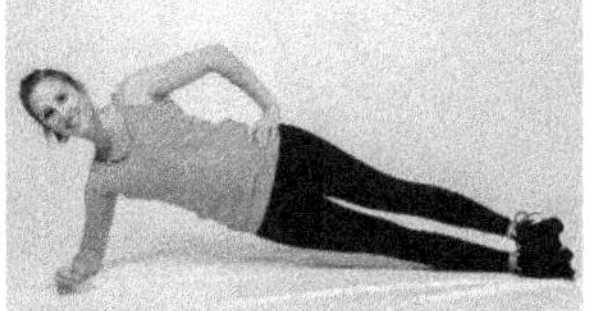

7.   1-minute rest. Repeat this circuit 2 more times for a total of 3 times. Once you have completed all three circuits put five minutes on your timer and stretch or perform yoga for that time. Really focus on elongating the body and relaxing the mind.

LD #4 perform each exercise for 30 seconds, rest when you need to, but try to complete an entire circuit before stopping. Ready to burn some fat? Let's go!!!

1.   Jog

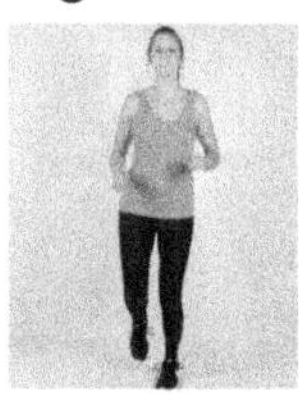 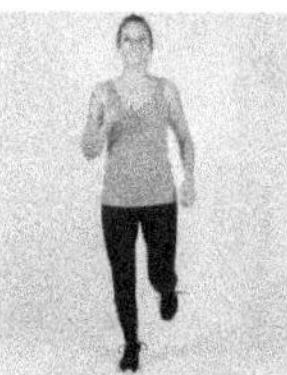

2.   Sumo Squats with Calf Raise

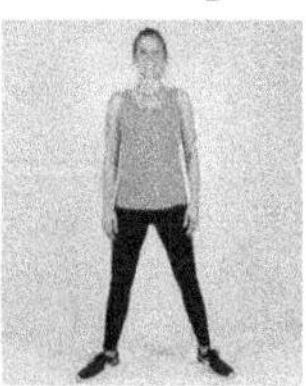 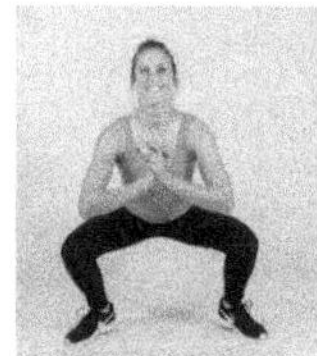 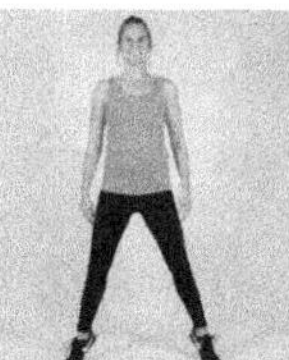

3.   Jog

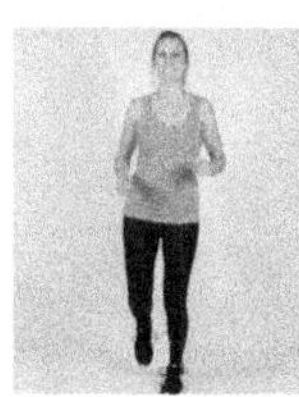 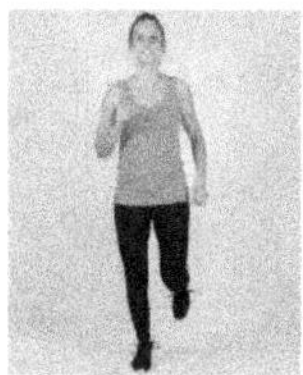

4.   Standard Calf Raise

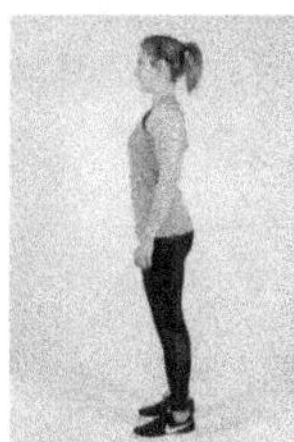 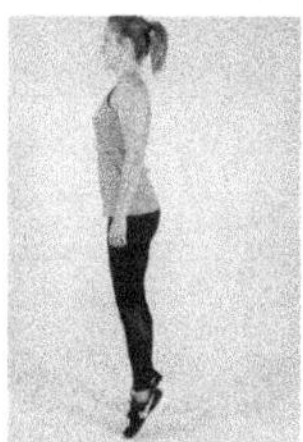

5.   Jog

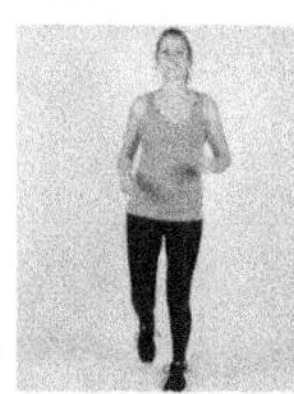 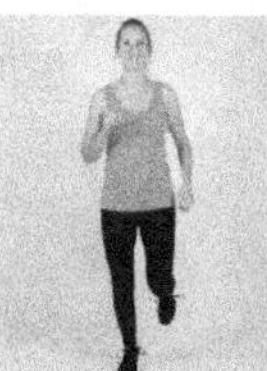

6.   Calf Raises with Toes Pointed Inward

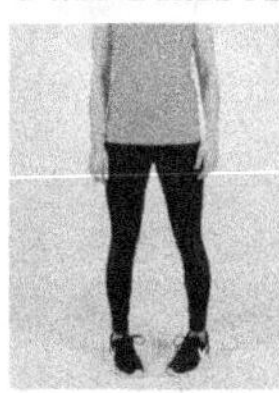 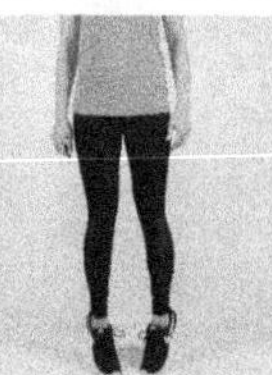

7.   1-minute rest. Repeat this circuit 2 more times for a total of 3 times. Once you have completed all three circuits put five minutes on your timer and stretch or perform yoga for that time. Really focus on elongating the body and relaxing the mind.

Fitness Dares

Every Saturday pick a new FD and learn there's more to "working out" than meets the eye

1. Sandy Toes

When you're on vacation, working out is typically not on your mind. This short, fast pace workout is a fun way to get the kids active and involved or get you motivated to get your sweat on! Have fun soaking up the sun and taking care of your body all at the same time. On a side note if you live in Alaska and are not on vacation nor are you on the beach you can still complete this workout as long as there is access to a pool. No pool? No worries, just skip the first exercises and move on to exercise 2.

- Swim 5 laps (if you're in a pool down and back= 1 lap).
- Measure and mark off 20 yards. Sprint down, then walk or jog back for 1. Complete in total, 5 sprints.
- Pulse squats for 60 seconds.
- Using the same distance as your sprints, complete 5 crab walks. Crab walk down the walk back to your starting line. If you don't know what a crab walk is, sit down on your bottom and then bridge up using your hands and feet. Then just walk backwards like a crab. Get the kiddos involved or your best friend and make it a race!
- 10 dolphin push-ups (see HD#3 on page 83 for model of exercise).
- Repeat this circuit 1 more time, for a total of 2 times.

2. Moving Mountains

Take a road trip with the family or go exploring in your neighborhood in search for the steepest hill or tallest set of stairs you can find. Complete 20 sprints up and walk back down. Next, to slow your heart rate down and to spend time with your family, walk around and have a scavenger hunt. See who can find the most treasures for the day. Whether you are with your kids, best friend, or spending quality time with your spouse just being in God's creation outside will fill your soul with happiness.

Treasure Hunt List

Coolest rock

Leaf

Feather

Berry

Flower

Something green

Something brown

Piece of trash (go throw it away afterwards)

Try to spot an animal

Look up and pick out a shape in the clouds

3. Random Act

Today is the day you get out of your comfort zone (if I haven't made you do that already) and try an extreme sport! (Or just a sport in general ha-ha). Go bike riding, snowboarding, surfing, kayaking, rock climbing. Go to an indoor jump park if it's raining or play a game of kickball with the neighborhood kids. Whatever you do today make it about family, fun, and getting a little sweaty. Like with everything in this book, it is all for the benefit and glory of God. If it wasn't for God loving us we would have no hope, but because that's not the case, we are going to spread a little love today. I want you at some point today to perform a random act of kindness. It could be paying for someone's food in the drive thru, helping someone load their groceries in the car, mow an elderly person's yard… the possibilities of showing love are endless! Go and get sweaty and let someone know they are loved today!

4. BFF Workout

Okay people grab up your best friend and go have fun together! This workout will require another person so recruit your BFF and let's get started!!! If you're not excited about working out today… misery loves company so grab your BFF and do it anyway! Do each exercise for 30 seconds with a 30 second break in-between.

- Planks with a high five- while facing one another plank, then give your friend a high five. You'll both be giving a high five with your right hands. Then rotate and do the left hands. You should be crossing your body each time with your arms.
- Wheelbarrows- grab your friends' ankles and let them walk on their hands. Let your friend push you around for 30 seconds then switch.
- Crunches with hand slaps- lay on your back with you and your friends toes touching. When you come up for a crunch you should be facing one another. Slap hands and come back keeping your belly button towards your spine. Complete 30 seconds.
- Commando crawls- while one friend is planking on their hands the other is commando crawling under. Once the friend crawling under is through, they will then plank and let the other friend commando crawl. Repeat this until 30 seconds are up.
- Back to back wall sits- using your friends back as a "wall" lock arms and sit back on one another till your legs are at 90 degrees. Hold pose for 30 seconds.
- Tandem bicycles- while laying on your backs put your feet against one another, raise your booty, and perform bicycles.
- Repeat these exercises 2 more times for a total of 3 times!

5. Park It

Be a kid again and go to your nearest park that has playground equipment. Instead of watching your little ones play while you sit on that park bench take this time to get a good sweat in.

- Go to the monkey bars and do pull-ups till fail. If you're unable to perform a pull-up go across the monkey bars until fail.
- Find something that isn't going to topple over or move (i.e. park bench, platform on the playground equipment etc.) and complete box jumps until fail.
- Going back to the monkey bars, hang on to the bars and while suspended perform knee raises to really target those lower abs.
- Find a set of stairs (or utilize that park bench again) and perform alternating step-ups.
- Walk or run 1 mile around the track field .
- Find a wall and do wall pushups until fail.
- Give yourself a nice little water break and let your heartrate go back down then repeat this workout 1 more time!

6. YC Day

Pick from one of the above workouts OR create your own workout routine to do for this day! Make sure you're getting in at least 30 minutes of exercise.

Recipes

Most of these recipes I have made up myself after trying to find ways to incorporate more healthy fats and vegetables into my family's meals. I encourage you to use my recipes and have fun with it! Add a little of this or that and make it your own. I find that when I'm creating something new I have much more fun in the kitchen than constantly looking at a recipe.

Some things to remember:
9g of sugar or less when purchasing items.
Homegrown or fresh is always better than the bought stuff.
I always cook in coconut oil unless otherwise stated.
I do not put serving sizes on these meals. You know your body and someone that weighs 115 lbs. and works a desk job will require less calories than someone that weights 165 lbs. and works in construction. Look on the labels and determine what a serving size looks like for you.

Turmeric Oatmeal

1. Cook one serving size of old fashioned oats per box directions. Once cooked add:

1 tbsp. nut butter
1 tbsp. honey
1 tsp turmeric
Dash of cinnamon
1 tbsp. flax seed

2. Mix well and serve.

Willingham Family Tradition

Pancakes, bacon or sausage, and eggs. My family has this same Sunday breakfast before church almost every Sunday.

Loaded Omelet

Egg (number of eggs depends on your body type and what you consider a serving size)
Cheese
Mushrooms
Peppers
Spinach
Ham

1. Mix everything together and cook in a greased pan (using coconut oil).

Chocolate Smoothie

1 frozen banana
¼ cup zucchini
½ cup strawberries
1 large tbl cacao powder
2 handfuls of spinach
2 tbl nut butter
1 tbl honey
2 tbl chia seeds
Dash of cinnamon
1 cup almond milk

1. Blend well and serve. You can also add ice if needed.

Blue-Bana Muffins

1 egg
3 very ripe bananas -mashed well
½ cup applesauce
½ cup blueberries
¼ cup chopped walnuts (optional)
¼ cup honey

3 tbl coconut oil
½ tbl cinnamon
1 tsp vanilla extract
1 tsp baking powder
½ tsp baking soda
¼ sea salt
1 ¼ cup gluten free flour

1. Preheat oven to 375 degrees F and spray your muffin pan.
2. With a blender, mix everything together except the flour and blueberries.
3. Add flour and blueberries and mix with a spoon (gently) until well combined.
4. Fill your muffin cups almost full and cook for 20-25 minutes or until a toothpick inserted in the middle comes out clean.
Note: I make a double batch and freeze the leftovers.

Peanut Butter Yogurt

4 oz Plain Greek Yogurt
1 tbs Peanut Butter (or Nut Butter of Choice)
1 tbs Honey
1 tsp Vanilla Extract
1 tsp Cinnamon

1. Mix together and serve.

Strawberry Banana Smoothie

1 frozen banana
1 cup strawberries (fresh or frozen)
1 handful of spinach
1tbl nut butter
2 tbl chia seeds
1cup almond milk
2 tbl honey
Dash cinnamon
¼ cup oats
1 tsp coconut oil

1. Combine, blend, serve.

Honey Toast

1-2 pieces GF bread
Honey
Cinnamon
Butter (or coconut oil)

1. Toast bread
2. Spread a small amount of butter over toast
3. Sprinkle cinnamon
4. Drizzle honey
5. Eat!
Note: you can also garnish with raisins.

Clean Pancakes

1 ripe banana
2 eggs
1 tsp cinnamon
1 tsp vanilla
1 tbl ground flax seed

1. Mash banana.
2. Beat eggs.
3. With a whisk or blender combine all ingredients very well.
4. Pour out desired amount onto a hot skillet and make pancakes. This will make 2-3 pancakes.

Avocado toast

1-2 slices of GF bread
½ Avocado
Red pepper flakes

1. Toast bread.
2. Spread avocado over toast.
3. Sprinkle red pepper flakes (if you like things spicy).

Nut Mix

½ cup walnuts ½ cup almonds   ¼ cup dried cranberries
¼ cup dark chocolate chips   ¼ cup oats

1. Mix together in an air tight container and serve.

Chef Salad

Spinach
Iceberg lettuce
Cubed ham
Cubed turkey
Cheddar cheese
Bacon
Boiled egg
Carrots
Bell pepper
Ranch dressing (or dressing of choice)

1. Toss everything together and serve.

Stuffed Peppers

12 oz. Italian sausage
3 large bell peppers, washed, cut in half lengthwise, and seeds removed (I like using a red, yellow, and orange. They seem to be more tender than the green ones, plus it's pretty.)
½ cup cooked brown rice
1 cup shredded cheddar cheese
1 can diced tomatoes and peppers (or fresh tomatoes and peppers diced)
2/3 cup of tomato juice (May need more or less depending on how thick you want it) I use homemade tomato juice but if you don't have fresh tomatoes you can always just take tomato sauce and water it down.

1. Crumble and cook sausage until brown.
2. Add rice, one can of diced tomatoes and peppers, tomato juice, and seasoning of your choice. I enjoy adding fresh herbs like parsley along with salt and pepper.
3. Bring to boil, then simmer about 10 minutes.
4. Take off heat and add half of your cheese.
5. Submerge peppers in boiling water for 5 minutes then remove and drain.
6. Place peppers in the same skillet as your sausage mixture and using a spoon, fill them with the mixture. It's okay if it spills out or it doesn't all fit in your peppers. Top with remaining cheese.
7. Pour more tomato juice around the peppers and bring to a boil, cover and simmer for about 10 minutes.
NOTE: This dish is awesome with a small side salad and an ear of corn! You can also substitute ground turkey or beef if you don't want Italian sausage.

Very Veggie Spaghetti

Packaged GF spaghetti noodles
16oz spaghetti sauce (make sure it has 9g of sugar or less)
1 lb. ground beef
1 carrot diced
½ small onion diced
3 cloves garlic pressed
½ small bell pepper diced
Handful of spinach, minced well
Parmesan and/or Romano cheese

1. Cook noodles per package directions.
2. While that's cooking sauté garlic and onion first for about 2 minutes.
3. Then add remaining vegetables and ground beef. Cook down until beef is browned and vegetables are tender. This is when I will salt and pepper everything well.
4. Add in spaghetti sauce and let simmer for 10 minutes.
5. Drain spaghetti.
6. Plate spaghetti, then sauce. Top with parmesan and Romano cheese and fresh parsley.

Chicken Caesar Salad

Romaine lettuce
Cooked grilled chicken breast
Parmesan cheese
Caesar dressing

1. Combine and serve. I add chia seeds on top for added crunch.

Shrimp Scampi Pasta

GF pasta of choice (cooked)
Pack of frozen pre-cooked shrimp (thawed)
Frozen broccoli (thawed)
3-4 cloves pressed garlic
Juice and zest of one lemon
Salt and pepper to taste
½ cup grated parmesan cheese
½ cup chicken stock
1. Add garlic, lemon, chicken stock, and parmesan cheese in a pan and simmer for about 5 minutes.
2. Add remaining ingredients and toss together.
3. Cover and simmer for about 3-5 minutes. Be careful not to overcook the shrimp.
4. Garnish with red pepper flakes if you like things spicy and enjoy!

Deer BBQ and Broccoli Slaw

Deer roast (you can obviously do beef or pork if preferred)
1 apple (cut in half)
1 onion (cut in half)
Celery seed
Ground mustard
2-3 bay dried bay leaves
Spices of your choice- if you like it spicy add cayenne, red pepper flakes, or fresh jalapenos
… if you like things sweet add 1 tbsp. of honey or maple syrup
BBQ sauce
Worcestershire sauce

1.Add roast and all ingredients into a crockpot. Cover with water and cook on low for
at least 6 hours.
2. Remove roast, let cool, and shred. Save some of the cooking juice.
3. Added shredded roast into a skillet and add cooking juice and BBQ sauce of choice.
Simmer for a few minutes and serve.
 NOTE: I purchase premade broccoli slaw and just use the recipe on the back of the packaging to make the slaw. Green beans also go well with this meal.

Chicken Avocado Burritos

Corn tortillas
Avocado
Shredded chicken
Ranch dressing
Mozzarella cheese

1. Put everything into tortilla, roll up, and cook on a griddle or sandwich press until cheese
has melted.

Shepherd's Pie

1 lb. ground beef	2 cups beef stock
11 oz. Frozen bag of mixed vegetables- thawed	2 tbl tomato paste
½ onion-diced	1 tbl worcestershire sauce
1 clove garlic- pressed	1 cup cheddar cheese
4 medium potatoes- peeled, cubed, and boiled	2 tbl butter
	Salt and pepper to taste (I also add some ground mustard and paprika

1. Heat oil and garlic in large skillet (I use cast iron), then sweat the onions.
2. Brown the meat.
3. Add tomato paste, worcestershire sauce, and beef stock. Let come to a boil then simmer for about 20 minutes.
4. Preheat oven to 350 degrees F.
5. Mash your boiled potatoes and butter together.
6. Add your thawed vegetables and mix well.
7. Then put on your potatoes onto the top of your dish until it's covered.
8. Add the cheese on top and place in the oven to cook for 20 minutes.
9. Let set for a few minutes before serving.

Baked Salmon

4-6 6oz salmon fillets
Zest and juice of 1 lemon
2 cloves of pressed garlic
2 tbl fresh herbs of choice (I prefer rosemary and parsley) finely minced
Salt and pepper
Paprika
1 tbl honey

1. Preheat oven broiler on high.
2. On a cookie sheet lay out aluminum foil.
3. Rub fish with the fresh herbs and garlic to coat.
4. Lay fish on foil and salt and pepper to taste.
5. Sprinkle paprika on fish.
6. Mix lemon juice and honey together and pour over fish.
7. Place under broiler for about 8-10 minutes until fish is cooked through. Then serve.
NOTE: if you prefer a not so lemony flavor then skip the zest and add 1-part lemon juice to 1-part honey along with about 2 tbl of water to dilute, then pour over fish.

Taco Salad

Lettuce
1lb. Grass Fed Ground Beef
Taco Seasoning
Corn Chips
Salsa
Sour Cream or Ranch Dressing
Shredded Cheddar Cheese

1. Brown meat and add seasoning into meat according to package. I make my own seasoning so I just eyeball this part and then add water to make it not so thick. If you also make your own, great! Play around with the amount till you get it perfect.
2. If you are making your own corn tortilla chips, this is the time to do that, if not then don't worry about this step, same goes with the salsa.
3. Assemble salad into a bowl and enjoy.

Turkey Chili

1 lb. ground turkey
Small onion
1 bell pepper
2 cloves garlic pressed
1 can kidney beans
1 can chili beans
1 small can tomato paste
1 can tomato sauce
1 tbl fresh minced parsley
2 tbl chili powder
1 tbl cumin powder
½ tbl. paprika
½ tbl ground mustard

1. In a large pot, sautee garlic, onions, and peppers.
2. Add turkey and cook until browned.
3. Add remaining ingredients and bring to a boil.
4. Cover and simmer for 30 minutes stirring often.
5. Watch and if it appears too thick add water. Typically, I always have to add water.
6. Garnish with corn chips, sour cream, and shredded cheese!
Hint: If you don't want to add all the spices or if you don't have them in your pantry, buy a premade chili spice packet. Just make sure it's gluten free.

Chicken or Pork and Roasted Vegetables

1. Cook the chicken/pork however you prefer. Sometimes I throw it on the grill, other times I bake it. Just decide what you're in the mood for. To make my roasted vegetables you'll need:

Your favorite type of vegetables
Coconut oil
Salt and pepper
Fresh rosemary

1. Preheat oven to 425 degrees F.
2. Wash and cube the vegetables. Normally, I'll use squash, zucchini, carrots, asparagus, and sweet potato.
3. Throw veggies into a large bowl and put salt, pepper, minced rosemary, and coconut oil.
4. With your hands mix until well-coated.
5. Put on a cookie tray and bake for 45 minutes.
6. Check the vegetables to see if they are soft, if not keep cooking for a few more minutes.
7. For an added bonus, you can sprinkle parmesan cheese on top of them and put back in the oven for 5 minutes or until the cheese has melted.

Cauliflower Pizza Crust

1 head of cauliflower (or 1 frozen bag)
1/3 cup crushed kale chips
½ tsp sea salt
½ tsp garlic powder
½ tsp dried oregano
2 eggs
½ shredded mozzarella cheese
1/3 cup grated parmesan cheese

1. Preheat oven to 425 degrees F and line a baking tray with parchment paper that has been lightly sprayed with cooking oil.
2. Rough chop your cauliflower and put in boiling water until a fork can by inserted into the vegetable with ease.
3. Drain and then blend in a food processor until the consistency of mashed potatoes has been reached.
4. Place mixture in a cheese cloth and squeeze all the water out. After you've squeezed out all the water you can let the mixture rest for 10 minutes then squeeze out again. The drier you can get the mixture the better.
5. Combine all ingredients in a mixing bowl and incorporate using a spoon.
6. Place dough onto baking tray and mash out to form a round pizza crust. Place in the oven and bake for 35-45 minutes.
7. Once cooled place toppings of choice and place back in the oven for about 10 minutes or until cheese has melted.
NOTE: you can also make this crust and freeze it for another time. It will keep in the freezer about 3 months.

Turkey Taco Bowl

1 lb. ground turkey
1 can black beans (drained)
1 can corn (drained)
1 cup water
1 package of taco seasoning
1 cup rice (cooked per package directions)

1. Brown turkey in a skillet then add taco seasoning, beans, corn, and cooked rice. Add water slowly until it reaches the right consistency of preference. I like mine to stick together but not be soupy. Simmer for about 15 minutes
2. Meanwhile prepare shredded lettuce, salsa, sour cream, cheese, and guacamole in separate bowls
3. Spoon out turkey into a bowl and top with prepared sides to make it your own. Enjoy!

Feta Salad

Spinach
Mixed greens (optional)
Feta cheese
Raspberry vinaigrette
Walnuts
Shredded chicken

1. Combine all ingredients and eat.
Note: this is a very light salad that will not weigh you down, but will definitely fill you up. Add more vegetables such as zucchini or peppers if you like. Remember to have fun with these recipes and make them your own.

No Bake Oatmeal Cookies

1 cup oats
¼ cup coconut oil
¼ cup peanut butter
¼ cup honey or maple syrup
Mini chocolate chips and pink Himalayan salt or sea salt for garnish

2 heaping tbsp. cacao powder
¼ tsp vanilla extract
1 tbl hemp seeds

1. Mix all ingredients together until all incorporated.
2. Spoon out onto wax paper and put in the freezer to chill for a few hours.
3. Eat whenever you need to satisfy that sweet tooth.
Hint: keep in the freezer because they melt very quickly.

Dark Chocolate Zucchini Muffins

2 eggs (whisked)
¾ cup nut butter
1/3 cup honey
¼ cup cacao powder
2 tbl GF pancake mix
1 tsp vanilla extract

1 tsp cinnamon
½ tsp nutmeg
Pinch of salt
1 cup chocolate chips
3 tbl almond milk (or whole milk)

1. Preheat oven to 375 degrees and line or grease cupcake pan.
2. Shred zucchini and remove excess water using a paper towel.
3. Mix together eggs, nut butter, and honey until combine and smooth.
4. Add remaining ingredients (except chocolate chips) and mix well.
5. Using a spoon fold chocolate chips into the batter.
6. Scoop batter into cupcake pan and bake for 25-35 minutes.

Avocado Fudge Brownie

1 ripe avocado
½ banana
¼ cup GF pancake mix
¼ cup cacao powder
½ cup honey
1 egg
½ cup chocolate chips

1. Preheat oven to 350 degrees.
2. In a food processor mix avocado and banana until smooth.
3. Combine remaining ingredients and blend until thoroughly incorporated .
4. Pour batter into a greased 9x9 baking dish and cook for 25-30 minutes.
5. Let cool and enjoy, these brownies store better when refrigerated.

Coco Nut Ice-Cream

1 or 2 frozen bananas
2 tbl peanut butter
1 tbl cacao powder
Toasted coconut and chocolate syrup

1. Using a food processor blend the frozen banana until thick and creamy.
2. Then add peanut butter and cacao powder, blend until fully combined.
3. Spoon out into a bowl and top with toasted coconut and chocolate syrup for a delicious refreshing treat.

Grocery List

Spices	Produce	Protein	Dairy	Grains/Seeds

Weekly Meal Plans

	Breakfast	Snack 1	Lunch	Snack 2	Supper
Monday					
Tuesday					
Wednesday					
Thursday					
Friday					
Saturday					
Sunday					

Weekly Workouts

Monday

Tuesday

Wednesday

Thursday

Friday

Saturday

Sunday

Roman Road to Salvation

For all have sinned and come short of the glory of God.
Romans 3:23

And for that, the wages of sin is death.
Romans 6:23

But the gift of God is eternal life through Jesus Christ our Lord.
Romans 6:23

But God commendeth His love toward us, in that, while we were yet sinners, Christ died for us.
Romans 5:8

For whosoever shall call upon the name of the Lord shall be saved.
Romans 10:13

That is thou shalt confess with thy mouth the Lord Jesus, and shalt believe in thine heart that God hath raised him from the dead, thou shalt be saved.
Romans 10:9

Present your bodies as a living sacrifice, holy, acceptable unto God, which is your reasonable service. And be not conformed to his world: but be ye transformed by the renewing of your mind, that ye may prove what is that good, and acceptable, and perfect, will of God.
Romans 12:1-2

9 781981 228522